Guide to Periodontics

D1336184

Guide to Periodontics

SECOND EDITION

W. M. M. JENKINS BDS, FDS, RCPS
Consultant in Periodontics,
Glasgow Dental Hospital and School.
Honorary Clinical Lecturer in Periodontology,
University of Glasgow.

C. J. ALLAN, BDS, FDS, RCPS
Consultant in Restorative Dentistry,
Dundee Dental Hospital and School.
Honorary Senior Lecturer in Periodontology,
University of Dundee.

and

W. J. N. COLLINS, BDS, MSc, FDS, RCPS
Director of Glasgow School of Dental Hygiene.
Honorary Clinical Lecturer in Periodontology,
University of Glasgow.

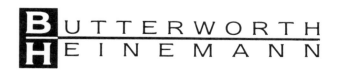

Butterworth-Heinemann Ltd
Linacre House, Jordan Hill, Oxford OX2 8DP

 PART OF REED INTERNATIONAL BOOKS

OXFORD   LONDON   BOSTON
MUNICH   NEW DELHI   SINGAPORE   SYDNEY
TOKYO   TORONTO   WELLINGTON

First published 1984
Reprinted 1986
Second edition 1988
Reprinted 1990, 1991, 1992

British Library Cataloguing in Publication Data
Jenkins, W. M. M.
    Guide to periodontics.–
    2nd ed.
    1. Dentistry. Periodontics.
    I. Title   II. Allan, C. J. (Christopher
    James), 1950–   III. Collins. W. J. N.
    (William John Nielson)

ISBN 0 7506 0267 8

Printed and bound in Great Britain by
Redwood Press Limited, Melksham, Wiltshire

Acknowledgements

Our sincere thanks and appreciation are extended to: Mr J. D.
Strahan and Dr Lars Heijl for reading the original manuscript
and for their helpful comments; Pamela Gibb for typing the
manuscripts; Ruth Swan and Anne Hughes for the drawings;
and Mr J. Davis and his staff in the Department of Dental
Illustration, Glasgow Dental Hospital and School, for the
photographic illustrations.

Contents

In writing this book our purpose has been to produce a concise text from which we hope the reader may obtain a sound perspective on periodontal disease and its treatment. It is not a manual of technique but rather an account of current practice in periodontics, and the concepts on which this is based. It is aimed primarily at the postgraduate who, having learned basic principles during undergraduate training, is reviving an interest in periodontology. We hope, also, that senior undergraduates will find it a useful adjunct to existing comprehensive textbooks.

The material has been carefully selected to allow us to develop the concepts upon which good clinical judgement is based. The first 17 chapters concern the biological basis and management of chronic periodontal disease. These are followed by one chapter on acute conditions and one on desquamative gingivitis.

We have made every effort to provide the reader with verifiable information although, rather than overwhelm him or her by including a large bibliography, we have cited only a few of the more useful publications. These include a number of review articles and some original research reports which expand the subject matter in areas less fully covered by our text. In this way it is hoped to stimulate the reader to further study.

In this second edition, the theme and general structure remain unaltered. Several chapters, however, have been rewritten and others changed to reflect recent developments in the specialty or to clarify and enlarge on the original material. A new chapter has been added describing recent research which we recognise as clinically important but which we feel is not yet sufficiently substantiated for routine application in clinical practice. A new appendix has been incorporated and the lists of recommended further reading have been updated. We trust that this second edition will continue to provide readers with a useful synopsis of current periodontal practice.

W. M. M. Jenkins
C. J. Allan
W. J. N. Collins

Chapter 1

Structure and Biology of the Periodontium

'Periodontium' is a term used to designate the functional structures which are directly involved in resisting forces applied to the teeth. These structures are the gingiva and supporting tissues (periodontal membrane, cementum and alveolar bone). The part of the periodontium which invests the coronal portion of the root is known as 'marginal periodontium'.

A full appreciation of the structure and biology of the periodontium can be obtained from standard periodontal textbooks. This chapter is limited to a brief description of the marginal periodontium, current knowledge of which is largely based on the excellent monograph of Schroeder and Listgarten first published in 1971 then revised in 1977.

GINGIVA

This is the fibrous mucosa surrounding the teeth and covering the coronal portion of the alveolar process (Figs. 1.1 and 1.2).

Attached Gingiva

This extends from the apical border of the free gingiva (*see below*) to the mucogingival junction, which separates the attached gingiva from the alveolar mucosa. The attached gingiva is pink in contrast to the deep red of alveolar mucosa. Attached gingiva is bound by dense bundles of collagen fibres to alveolar bone and, further coronally, to the root cementum forming the supracrestal fibre attachment. It is lined by oral epithelium which is stratified squamous and keratinised with rete peg formations. There is great variation in width of attached gingiva. It is usually widest (6·0 mm) on the lingual aspect of the first molar region of the mandible, and narrowest (0·5 mm) on the buccal aspect of the third molar region of the mandible. In the palate, there is no clear demarcation between the attached gingiva and palatal

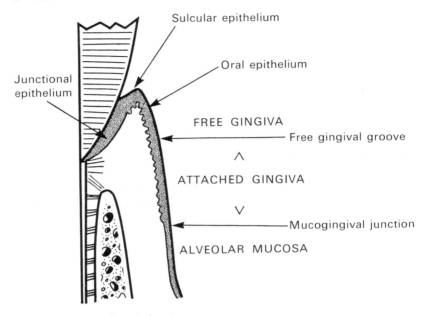

Fig. 1.1   *Marginal periodontium.*

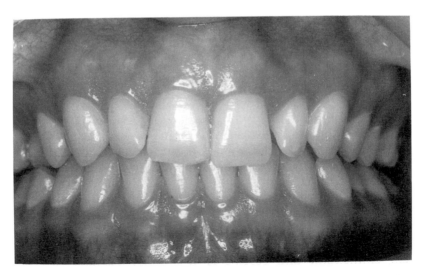

Fig. 1.2   *Clinical appearance of normal gingiva: the gingiva has a 'knife-edge' margin coronal to the amelocemental junction; 'stippling' is apparent in some areas.*

mucosa, both of which are keratinised structures. As attrition or loss of opposing teeth occurs, compensatory over-eruption may take place, increasing the width of attached gingiva, the mucogingival junction being static while the gingival margin maintains its relationship to the tooth by moving coronally with it.

Free Gingiva

This consists of the marginal part of the gingiva which can be deflected from the tooth surface by a probe inserted into the gingival sulcus. Anatomically, the apical boundary of the free gingiva is usually regarded as the free gingival groove, a shallow linear depression on the outer surface of the gingiva, parallel to the gingival margin, but found in only one-third of persons with normal gingiva. When present, therefore, the free gingival groove represents, on the outer surface of the gingiva, the probing depth of the gingival sulcus.

Interdentally, the free gingiva extends to the contact point and forms the interdental papilla. Immediately below the contact point there is a slight depression, saddle or 'col'. The broader contact area of posterior teeth is associated with a larger col and separate buccal, and lingual papillae may be recognised. For descriptive purposes, the free gingiva is sometimes subdivided into marginal gingiva, lining the buccal and lingual surfaces, and papillary gingiva, interdentally.

The epithelium of the free gingiva may be divided into three morphologically distinct compartments, and these are described below.

Oral epithelium. This is continuous with the epithelial lining of attached gingiva. It extends up to the gingival margin but not into the sulcus. It resembles the epithelium of attached gingiva—stratified squamous and keratinised with rete peg formation.

Sulcular (crevicular or oral sulcular) epithelium. This is continuous with, and structurally similar to, the oral epithelium of the gingiva. It is not, however, keratinised. Below the contact point of adjacent teeth the sulcular epithelium is continuous with col epithelium, and resembles it closely. Sulcular and col epithelia are closely related to the tooth surface but are not attached to it. In health the gingival sulcus (crevice) is about 0·5 mm deep histologically although, with perfect chemical

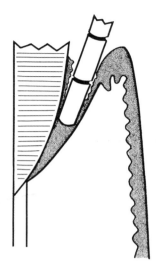
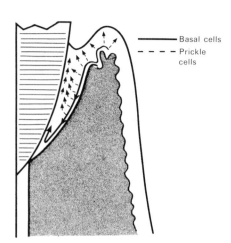

Basal cells
- - - - Prickle
cells

Fig. 1.3 *Probing a healthy sulcus.*

Fig. 1.4 *Epithelial cell migration in gingival epithelium. The continuous line indicates how the basal layer of junctional epithelium is repopulated after wounding.*

plaque control and in the absence of irritant effects of mechanical cleansing procedures, its depth approaches zero. Clinically, rather greater sulcus depths of 1–2 mm are detected by probing as the probe tip passes into the junctional epithelium (Fig. 1.3).

Junctional epithelium. This is the epithelial collar which extends apically from the base of the sulcus to the amelocemental junction—a distance of about 2·5 mm. It is derived from reduced enamel epithelium and replenished by oral epithelium. The cells of the junctional epithelium are loosely knit, with wide intercellular spaces. Keratinisation does not take place. The epithelial–connective tissue interface is smooth and rete pegs are not found. At the dentogingival junction the junctional epithelium forms an attachment, 'the epithelial attachment', to the tooth surface. The epithelial attachment apparatus is synthesised by the epithelium itself and consists of a basement lamina and hemidesmosomes. This form of attachment is very dynamic, allowing coronal movement of epithelial cells and their eventual desquamation into the gingival sulcus (Fig. 1.4).

Although structurally different, the junctional, sulcular and oral epithelia are formed of cells which are fundamentally similar but which adapt to a specific environment created by the tone of underlying collagen fibres and blood pressure. These factors determine the amount of contact which the epithelium makes against the tooth surface. Following gingivectomy, a covering of epithelium will form by coronal migration of cells from the wound margin, and this will assume the characteristic features of junctional, sulcular and oral epithelia.

SUPPORTING TISSUES

In health, the alveolar bone crest on the approximal surface lies 1·0 mm apical to the amelocemental junction. On buccal and lingual surfaces, however, depending on tooth position and inclination, this distance may be considerably greater, amounting in some cases to a dehiscence. In this situation, a longer supracrestal fibre attachment is present. The periodontal membrane (ligament) attaches the tooth to alveolar bone. The reader is referred to Berkovitz *et al.* (1982) for a comprehensive study of the periodontal ligament.

The cells of the periodontal ligament have a unique property. Following treatment of a previously diseased root surface these cells alone have the potential to form new cementum and periodontal ligament. This ability, however, would manifest itself only if bone, gingival epithelium and gingival connective tissue could be prevented from occupying the surface of the root within the wound area during healing. In fact, with current therapeutic techniques, rapid proliferation of gingival epithelium invariably occurs, resulting in an *epithelial* attachment.

DEFENCE MECHANISMS OF THE GINGIVAL SULCUS

Gingival (sulcular, crevicular) fluid is an exudate, present in small amounts in health and in much larger quantities when inflammation is clinically apparent. Gingival fluid reaches the sulcus via the junctional epithelium, mixing with polymorphonuclear neutrophilic granulocytes (neutrophils) and, to a lesser extent, monocytes which migrate by the same route as a result of chemotaxis from bacterial products.

The formation of bacterial plaque close to the gingival margin is a continuous process interrupted only briefly by oral hygiene procedures and the dentogingival junction represents a potential entry for toxic bacterial products reaching the underlying connective tissue. Periodontal health is maintained to some extent by:

a)   the anatomical epithelial seal preventing bacteria in the gingival sulcus from reaching the connective tissue;
b)   dynamic shedding of degenerated and infected junctional epithelial cells from the base of the sulcus;
c)   rapid repair of junctional epithelium following injury;
d)   flushing effect of gingival fluid;
e)   the constant stream of neutrophils, migrating through junctional epithelium into the gingival sulcus.

REFERENCES

Berkovitz B. K. B., Moxham B. J., Newman H. N. eds. (1982). *The Periodontal Ligament in Health and Disease.* Oxford: Pergamon Press.

Schroeder H. E., Listgarten M. A. (1977). Fine structure of the developing epithelial attachment of human teeth. *Monographs of Developmental Biology*, Vol. 2, 2nd edn. Basel: S. Karger.

Chapter 2

Pathogenesis

DEFINITIONS

Periodontal disease

This term, in its widest sense, includes all pathological conditions of the periodontium. It is, however, commonly used with reference to those inflammatory diseases which are plaque-induced and which affect the marginal periodontium: gingivitis and periodontitis.

Gingivitis. This is an inflammatory response of the gingiva without destruction of supporting tissues. The commonest form of gingival disease is chronic gingivitis, caused by bacterial plaque. In chronic gingivitis, gingival enlargement and loss of resistance to probing occur. A gingival pocket may be present.

Periodontitis. This term describes a group of inflammatory diseases affecting all the periodontal structures, of which the commonest is chronic adult periodontitis. Periodontitis results from an apical extension of the inflammatory process, initiated in the gingiva. Destruction of the periodontal attachment results in a periodontal pocket.

DEVELOPMENT OF CHRONIC GINGIVITIS
(Fig. 2.1(a)–(c))

There is no clear dividing line between gingival health and gingivitis either in clinical or histopathological terms. Even gingiva that appears clinically healthy will exhibit a small inflammatory infiltrate.

When plaque is allowed to accumulate freely there is an acute exudative inflammatory response within two to four days. This response occurs in the connective tissue subjacent to the coronal portion of the junctional epithelium (Fig. 2.1(a)). The changes include vasculitis, perivascular collagen destruction, enhanced production of gingival fluid and an increase in neutrophil migration into the junctional epithelium. At this stage, however,

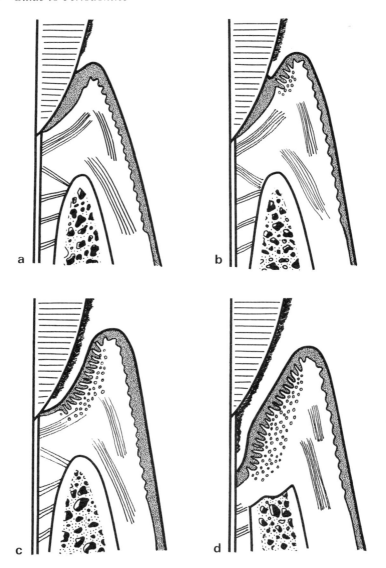

Fig. 2.1   *The development of chronic gingivitis and periodontitis. (a) A healthy gingival sulcus with early supragingival plaque formation. (b) Established chronic gingivitis with minor inflammatory enlargement. (c) Long-standing chronic gingivitis with subgingival plaque extension in a gingival pocket. (d) Chronic periodontitis with destruction of periodontal membrane and alveolar bone and apical migration of epithelial attachment.*

there is no change in clinical appearance. After four to seven days, as the acute exudative response persists, the connective tissues are infiltrated by T-lymphocytes. After 10–21 days of persistent plaque accumulation, further evidence of an immune response is apparent as plasma cells emerge within the cellular infiltrate. Chronic inflammatory cells now overshadow the acute exudative response. Further collagen loss occurs. This stage is described as established chronic gingivitis (Fig. 2.1(b)). A shallow gingival pocket may be evident and bleeding may occur in response to probing. In due course, the cellular infiltrate becomes dominated by plasma cells.

Gingivitis is initiated by supragingival plaque accumulation but, as gingival enlargement occurs, a subgingival flora is created. Apical advancement of subgingival plaque occurs at a later stage, the junctional epithelium becoming detached from the tooth surface to become pocket epithelium. This is characterised by the formation and extension of rete pegs with microscopic areas of ulceration between them (Fig. 2.1(c)).

Although collagen destruction always takes place within the marginal gingiva adjacent to the tooth surface, in long-standing gingivitis there may be proliferative activity by fibroblasts outside the infiltrated zone, nearer the oral surface of the gingiva. This results in fibrous gingival enlargement and masks the underlying inflammation.

CLINICAL FEATURES OF CHRONIC GINGIVITIS
(Fig. 2.2)

Marginal redness. The degree of erythema depends on the intensity of the inflammatory response as well as the bucco-lingual thickness and consistency of gingival tissue. 'Thick' fibrotic gingival tissue will conceal the inflammation present on its inner surface.

Bleeding on probing. This occurs when the friable pocket lining with its underlying dilated vasculature is traumatised. Bleeding on probing often precedes visual signs of inflammation such as redness or swelling.

Swelling. Blunting of interdental papillae and thickening of the free gingival margin is a result of oedema and/or a reactive increase in tissue cells (hyperplasia).

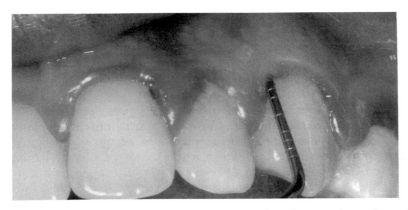

Fig. 2.2   *Chronic gingivitis. There is marginal oedema, redness, loss of contour and bleeding on probing.*

Loss of stippling. This is a variable phenomenon, thought to be caused by the accumulation of oedema fluid.

Increased probing depth. The inflammatory reaction will result in gingival enlargement and/or loss of resistance to probing, both giving rise to an increased probing depth beyond the norm of 1–2 mm.

Severity

Generally, in individuals with a normal host response to plaque, the severity of gingivitis simply reflects the level of plaque control. However, complex forms of gingivitis exist where the tissue response is exaggerated by an underlying local or systemic modifying factor and these individuals may exhibit a level of gingivitis not commensurate with the quantity of plaque. Some of these conditions have specific clinical or histopathological features which differentiate them from simple gingivitis (*see* Chapter 3 *and* Appendix III).

THE TRANSITION STAGE

Although gingivitis can develop quickly (within 10–21 days following withdrawal of plaque control measures), an equilibrium is usually established between the increased mass of bacteria and the host defences, maintaining a state of chronic gingivitis indefinitely. The transition from gingivitis to perio-dontitis may occur at any time. If and when it does occur, it is assumed to involve an imbalance in the host–parasite equilibrium. This imbalance may be precipitated either by a proportional increase in pathogenic organisms within the sub-gingival microflora or impaired host resistance, or by both factors in combination. While it is thought that gingivitis is a necessary precursor to periodontitis, some individuals may develop periodontitis without evidence of gross marginal gingivitis. This supports the idea that gingivitis and periodontitis are separate diseases with different host–parasite interactions.

DEVELOPMENT OF CHRONIC PERIODONTITIS
(Fig. 2.1(d))

As soon as the destructive process within the marginal gingiva extends apically to affect the collagen fibre attachment of the root surface, gingivitis becomes periodontitis. The further apical extension of the inflammatory process is thought to proceed in a series of 'bursts' of destructive activity interspersed with periods of quiescence representing temporary re-establishment of the host–parasite equilibrium.

The nature of the destructive process in chronic periodontitis is described below. It includes all the features of established gingivitis, i.e. a predominantly plasma cell infiltrate with various acute inflammatory alterations. It is preferable to think of the following events (a–e) as occurring simultaneously rather than in sequence. It will be noted that while features (a) and (b) occur also to a limited extent in the later stages of gingivitis, (c–e) are specific to periodontitis.

a) Apical advancement of subgingival plaque.
b) The coronal portion of junctional epithelium, as it is separated from the tooth surface by bacterial plaque, becomes transformed into 'pocket epithelium'.
c) Inflammatory changes subjacent to the pocket epithelium and the residual junctional epithelium are accompanied by the destruction of gingival connective tissue, periodontal membrane and alveolar bone. Shallow resorptive lesions of cementum may occur.
d) Destruction of the collagen fibre attachment apical to the

junctional epithelium enables it to proliferate apically on the root surface. A strand of junctional epithelium will always be present at the base of the advancing pocket, denying the bacteria access to the connective tissues in this direction. The apical migration of junctional epithelium in this way results in 'migration of epithelial attachment'.

e)   As subgingival plaque extends onto the root surface, the cementum may adsorb plaque endotoxins. These plaque endotoxins may have an irritant effect on the overlying soft tissue, preventing repair, unless the surface layers of cementum are removed along with plaque and calculus deposits during treatment.

CLINICAL FEATURES OF CHRONIC PERIODONTITIS
(Figs. 2.3, 2.4)

The formation of pathological pockets is common to both gingivitis and periodontitis. The distinguishing feature of periodontitis is 'loss of connective tissue attachment'. In theory, this can be assessed clinically by measuring with a probe the distance between the amelocemental junction and the base of the pocket. Accurate measurement of attachment levels depends on the ability of the probe to 'split' the junctional epithelium and penetrate to the most coronally attached fibres. In fact, healthy gingival tissues will resist probing pressure while inflammation at the base of the pocket may allow the probe tip to penetrate the connective tissue. Clinical attachment-level recordings are, thereby, subject to a small measurement error. The exact amount of attachment loss can be determined only by histology.

Periodontal pockets, once formed, will persist indefinitely unless they are treated. On the other hand, continuous destruction is by no means inevitable. It would appear that, in some cases, progressive loss of attachment ceases for extended periods of time, perhaps even permanently. In other individuals, or at other tooth sites, the destruction may be intermittent, periods of exacerbation being interspersed with periods of remission and repair.

Periodontitis is detected most readily with a probe, a blood-stained or purulent exudate being elicited by probing to the base of the pocket beyond the amelocemental junction (Fig. 2.3). It must be stressed that bleeding from the base of the pocket

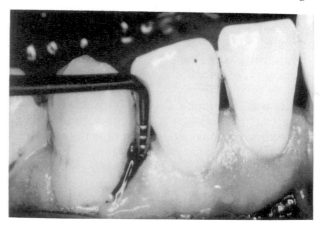

Fig. 2.3 *Advanced chronic periodontitis in the absence of readily detectable gingival changes: the probe as an essential diagnostic tool.*

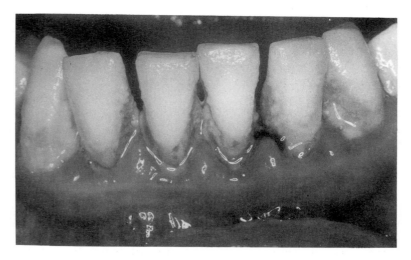

Fig. 2.4 *Advanced chronic periodontitis. Gingival recession, tooth migration and mobility are present while marginal gingivitis persists owing to poor oral hygiene.*

on probing merely denotes inflammation; it is not a sign of *active* destruction. In other words, bleeding on probing is likely to occur during periods of remission as well as during progressive destruction.

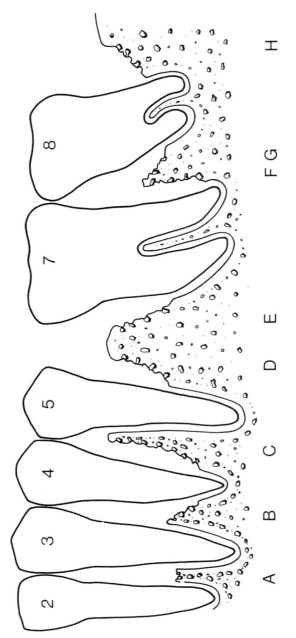

Fig 2.5   *Two-dimensional image of interdental bone defects A–H, which could originate as follows. A. The interdental septum is less than 2 mm wide: horizontal bone loss could arise from apical extension of plaque on one or both roots. B. Bone loss on coronal half of $\overline{3}$ where interdental septum is less than 2 mm wide could be due to apical extension of plaque on $\overline{3}$ and $\overline{4}$ or $\overline{4}$ alone. Angular defect on mesial of $\overline{4}$ signifies more rapid disease progress on $\overline{4}$ than $\overline{3}$. C. Broad interdental septum: mesial of $\overline{5}$ is not affected by periodontitis. D, E. Very wide interdental bone allowing two separate angular defects. F, G. Interdental septum broad enough apically to allow separate angular defects after narrower crestal bone totally destroyed. H. Very wide bone defect. Resorbed surface outside radius of action of tooth-associated plaque, but could be caused either by subsequent mesial drift or bacterial invasion of pocket wall.*

Patterns of Bone Destruction

Bone destruction goes hand in hand with loss of connective tissue attachment and is essentially a *locally* destructive process, usually confined to a zone up to about 2 mm wide along the affected root surface. Bone outside this zone lies beyond the effective radius of action of subgingival plaque. Thus, where the alveolar housing is thin, on buccal and lingual aspects and interdentally towards the necks of teeth, the apical extension of plaque will lead to destruction of the entire thickness of the alveolar process. This is so-called 'horizontal bone loss'. Frequently interdental bone, and less often buccal or lingual bone, is thicker than 2 mm so that resorption affects only the portion of bone lining the affected tooth surface with the formation of an 'angular' or 'vertical' bone defect. Thus the pattern of bone destruction within the mouth and around individual teeth reflects differences in bone morphology as well as the quantity and pathogenicity of plaque and its interaction with host defences. This theory is based on the work of Waerhaug (1979*a*, *b*) and Fig. 2.5 illustrates how it may be applied to explain interdental bone resorption.

Suprabony pockets. These are pockets which do not extend apical to the adjacent alveolar crest (Fig. 2.1(d)). These pockets develop in association with horizontal bone loss, i.e. resorption of the entire thickness of the alveolar process.

Infrabony pockets. These are pockets which extend apical to the adjacent alveolar crest (note that the term '*intra*bony' is preferred by some authors but is reserved by others to describe a three-walled infrabony pocket). Infrabony pockets are always associated with an angular bone defect and are usually classified according to the number of bone walls which surround the pocket. Figure 2.6 illustrates some of the many possible configurations. One of the commonest types of defect, the 'interdental crater' is illustrated separately in Fig. 2.7 (the buccal and lingual walls form the sides of two two-walled pockets on adjacent proximal surfaces). This classification, while good in theory, is difficult to apply since most infrabony pockets taper towards their bases retaining additional 'bone walls' in the process. For treatment purposes, three-walled pockets are preferred since these show the greatest potential for bone-fill. At the opposite extreme a one-walled 'hemiseptum' defect with a broad opening offers a poor framework for bone-fill, and

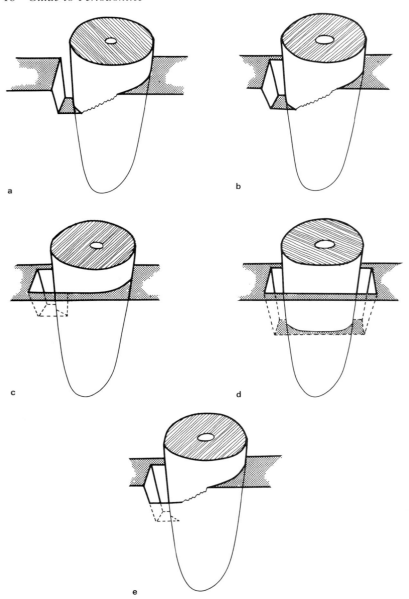

Fig. 2.6   *Angular bone defects:* (a) *one approximal bone wall (hemiseptum),*
(b) *two walls,* (c) *three walls,* (d) *four walls (funnel defect),* (e) *two
walls coronally, three walls apically.* (c) *and* (d) *have good potential
for bone-fill;* (b) *and* (e) *have rather less potential for bone-fill.*

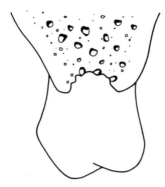

Fig. 2.7 *Two-walled defect: interdental crater.*

attempts to eliminate the defect by bone resection would damage the support of the less affected adjacent tooth.

Complicating Factors

Furcation lesions, periodontal–pulpal disease, gingival recession, tooth migration and hypermobility are all pathological features of advancing chronic periodontitis (Fig. 2.4) and are dealt with in detail in Chapters 11, 12, 13 and 15.

Terminal Periodontitis

Untreated periodontitis may eventually give rise to acute painful episodes or culminate in exfoliation. The former may present as an acute periodontal abscess or as pulpitis due to toxic substances reaching the pulp from plaque deposits on the root surface. Pulp necrosis may also occur when apical vessels are affected by occlusal trauma in cases of advanced loss of supporting tissue. Although such changes do not preclude attempts at treatment, they are usually indicative of deep-seated disease when extraction may be unavoidable.

REFERENCES

Waerhaug J. (1979*a*). The angular bone defect and its relationship to trauma from occlusion and downgrowth of sub-gingival plaque. *Journal of Clinical Periodontology*; 6: 61–82.

Waerhaug J. (1979*b*). The infrabony pocket and its relationship to trauma from occlusion and sub-gingival plaque. *Journal of Periodontology*; 50: 355–65.

FURTHER READING

Dolby A. E. (1980). Host response to dental bacterial plaque. In *Efficacy of Treatment Procedures in Periodontics*. (Shanley D., ed.) p. 197. Chicago: Quintessence.

Listgarten M. A. (1986). Pathogenesis of periodontitis. *Journal of Clinical Periodontology*; 13: 418–25.

Page R. C. (1986). Gingivitis. *Journal of Clinical Periodontology*; 13: 345–55.

Page R. C., Schroeder H. E. (1981). Current status of the host response in chronic marginal periodontitis. *Journal of Periodontology*; 52: 477–91.

Schroeder H. E., Attstrom R. (1980). Pocket formation: An hypothesis. In *The Borderland between Caries and Periodontal Disease, II*. pp. 99–123. London: Academic Press.

Socransky S. S., Haffajee A. D., Goodson J. M., Lindhe J. (1984). New concepts of destructive periodontal disease. *Journal of Clinical Periodontology*; 11: 21–32.

Chapter 3

Aetiology

Periodontal disease is initiated and maintained by bacterial plaque. The extent of tissue damage is dependent on the interaction between plaque bacteria and host defence mechanisms. Local environmental factors may favour the accumulation of bacterial plaque. Systemic or local modifying factors act by altering the host response to bacterial plaque.

THE INITIATING FACTOR — DENTAL BACTERIAL PLAQUE

The earliest deposit to form on a cleaned tooth surface is the acquired pellicle—a structureless film of salivary glycoproteins selectively adsorbed on to hydroxyapatite crystals. It forms within minutes of a polish with pumice. After three or four hours, colonies of Gram-positive coccoid bacteria are found on the tooth surface both supragingivally and within the gingival sulcus. These bacteria belong mainly to the genus *Streptococcus*. A wide range of other micro-organisms can be found, but mostly in small numbers. If plaque accumulation continues uninterrupted for 10–21 days, during which time inconsistent changes in microbial composition may be noted, frank gingivitis develops. Generally, *Actinomyces* species and Gram-negative rods constitute a larger proportion of the microflora as gingivitis develops, but such is the variation from subject to subject and site to site that the specific presence of these organisms is not believed to be of aetiological significance. Gingivitis is therefore associated mainly with quantitative changes in bacterial plaque rather than the overgrowth of specific micro-organisms.

Like gingivitis, periodontitis is caused by plaque, by subgingival down-growth of those bacteria best able to evade host defences and survive in a low-oxygen environment. The composition of subgingival plaque, therefore, differs from that of plaque on the adjacent visible tooth surfaces. For example, in subgingival plaque, Gram-positive bacteria are found in lower proportions and Gram-negative bacteria in higher proportions than in supragingival plaque. The subgingival flora comprises a layer of tooth-attached plaque as well as a loosely adherent component in direct association with the pocket epithelium. The tooth-attached plaque consists mainly of Gram-positive rods and cocci while the unattached plaque contains a predominance of Gram-negative organisms including motile forms. The relatively stagnant environment of the pocket will encourage the colonisation of those bacteria not readily able to adhere to the tooth surface. Motile organisms, therefore, will be found in higher proportions within loosely adherent subgingival plaque than anywhere else in the mouth.

Those organisms thought to be of greatest aetiological significance in periodontitis are listed in Chapter 20 (Table 20.1), which contains a more detailed discussion of the microbial aetiology of periodontitis.

The mechanisms by which bacteria may provoke an inflammatory response and cause tissue destruction are complex. Bacteria themselves generally do not penetrate junctional epithelium. However, various substances produced by bacteria (endotoxin, mucopeptides, lipoteichoic acids, metabolic products, proteolytic agents, hyaluronidase and chondroitinase) will penetrate and infiltrate the gingival tissues, causing direct injury. Bacteria may also act indirectly by triggering host-mediated responses which may result in self-injury. The gingival fluid, which is produced at all stages and in all forms of periodontal disease, as well as having defensive properties, contains growth factors for a number of bacteria, facilitating more rapid plaque accumulation. Accordingly, more frequent oral hygiene practices will be required to resolve than to prevent gingivitis.

A subgingival flora, once established, will persist in spite of improved supragingival plaque control. Furthermore, subgingival débridement will be successful in producing a physiological gingival sulcus only if it results in a sufficiently plaque-free environment to allow repair to take place. With pockets over 3 mm, there is an increasing likelihood that some bacterial deposits will remain, to recolonise the subgingival environment and perpetuate the inflammatory lesion.

HOST DEFENCE MECHANISMS

The host defence system is made up of local tissue components, together with eosinophils, basophils and mast cells, neutrophils and monocytes, the immune response and serum factors such as the complement system. The activities of these host defence mechanisms would appear to be both protective and destructive, and in most cases the tissue damage sustained is minor relative to the protection provided. An intact and normally functioning host response would appear to be compatible with, at worst, slowly progressive periodontal disease. However, changes in the capacity of various components of the host response to deal with the bacterial challenge may alter the characteristics of periodontal disease. For example, abnormalities in neutrophil or monocyte function have been associated with rapidly destructive disease.

LOCAL ENVIRONMENTAL FACTORS

Calculus

Mineralisation within plaque results in calculus formation. Calcification may commence within 24 hours of plaque accumulation but the rate of formation is very variable between individuals. Subgingival calculus forms more slowly and, being firmly attached, is usually more difficult to remove. Calculus is always covered by plaque and retains toxic bacterial products. The removal of calculus is, therefore, of fundamental importance in periodontal treatment.

Dental Morphological Factors

The palatal groove, occasionally present on upper incisors, may be an ideal place for plaque to accumulate and cause a narrow but rapidly destructive lesion of the periodontium. Likewise, plaque may accumulate undisturbed in the mesial fossa of the upper first premolar, just apical to the contact point.

Soft-Tissue Factors

The presence of a fraenum, attached close to the gingival margin, may impede satisfactory plaque control, as may a shallow vestibule (*see* Chapter 13).

Crowding

Crowded, malpositioned teeth may present difficulties in plaque control, and access for scaling procedures may be restricted.

Restorations and Prostheses

This will be described in greater detail in Chapter 17. Restorative materials, with the exception of glazed porcelain, accumulate plaque more rapidly than intact enamel. Unpolished or unglazed restorations will accumulate plaque more readily. Poor crown and pontic contour, especially excessive axial contours, favour plaque retention near the gingival margin. Above all, subgingival restorations, especially those with defective or overhanging margins, may have a profound effect on periodontal health by retaining plaque within a gingival pocket. Partial-denture wearers will accumulate more dental bacterial plaque because of impaired natural cleansing.

SYSTEMIC MODIFYING FACTORS

A number of systemic disorders have been shown to increase the severity of plaque-induced periodontal diseases. Examples are listed below.

Pregnancy

It is well established that there is an increase in severity of gingivitis during pregnancy until the eighth month, when the severity of gingivitis begins to decline. The gingival changes are thought to be caused by the effect of increased levels of progesterone on the microvasculature. Apart from generalised gingival changes, a pregnancy granuloma may occur (Fig. 3.1). This hyperplastic lesion has the same histology as the 'pyogenic granuloma'. Newly formed capillaries dominate the lesion.

Puberty

Hormonal imbalance is considered by some to be a cause of the increased severity of gingivitis witnessed at puberty. On the other hand, the peak at this age group may be attributed to an increase

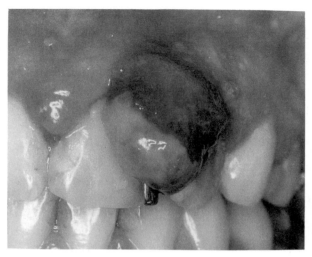

Fig 3.1 *Ulcerated pregnancy epulis. This lesion reveals the concurrence of the initiating factor (plaque) with a local environmental factor (overhanging cervical margin of the gold inlay in [1]) and a systemic modifying factor (pregnancy).*

in gingival sites at risk as the permanent dentition develops and to improved oral hygiene after puberty resulting from increased social awareness.

Diabetes Mellitus

Deficient neutrophil chemotaxis and phagocytosis together with depressed macrophage activity may account for the reported increase in severity of gingivitis and periodontitis in diabetics. This association is more likely to be observed in poorly controlled individuals.

Blood Dyscrasias

Agranulocytosis and neutropenia. Agranulocytosis and neutropenia, including cyclic neutropenia, are associated with an increased severity of gingivitis, necrotic ulceration and advanced periodontal destruction.

Acute leukaemia. Gingival enlargement, ulceration, inflammation, purpura and severe bleeding are characteristic of some cases of acute leukaemia attributable to the infiltration of malignant cells, neutropenia, impaired phagocytosis, platelet deficiency and decreased effectiveness of immune mechanisms. If the patient survives long enough, advanced periodontal destruction may also be noted. Cytotoxic drugs and antibiotics may have a variety of adverse or beneficial effects on the clinical periodontal picture.

Hereditary and Genetic Factors

Hereditary gingival fibromatosis is a rare condition, possibly transmitted by a dominant gene, where there is often gross fibrous enlargement of the gingiva in response to plaque accumulation. Affected individuals are usually otherwise healthy.

Down's syndrome may be associated with greater severity of periodontal disease, perhaps due to altered connective tissue metabolism.

Hyperkeratosis palmaris et plantaris (Papillon-Lefèvre syndrome), hypophosphatasia and Chediak-Higashi syndrome are rare conditions associated with rapidly destructive plaque-induced periodontal disease. Chediak-Higashi syndrome is characterised by defective neutrophils.

Drug Ingestion

Oral contraceptive drugs have been shown to cause an increased severity of gingivitis and, after prolonged use, greater loss of attachment.

The antiepileptic drug phenytoin is a well-known cause of fibrous gingival hyperplasia. It affects about 50% of individuals taking the drug. The severity of the gingival reaction is related both to the dosage and to the level of oral hygiene. There is no satisfactory evidence that phenytoin can exhibit its effect in the absence of local irritants.

More recently, it has been shown that severe fibrous gingival hyperplasia can be caused by cyclosporin-A and nifedipine. Cyclosporin-A is an immunosuppressant drug used primarily in organ transplantation. Nifedipine is a relatively new peripheral and coronary vasodilator which is used in the treatment of angina pectoris and hypertension.

LOCAL MODIFYING FACTORS

Lip-apart Posture

Gingival tissue will often respond adversely to an incompetent lip seal with marked erythema of the free and attached gingiva and inflammatory enlargement. This is indisputable. The mechanism for these changes, however, is not well understood. The upper anterior teeth will not be fully exposed to salivary antimicrobial agents, which, together with lack of functional cleaning, may result in increased plaque accumulation and, therefore, increased gingivitis. Furthermore, even in the absence of plaque, drying of the gingiva is likely to result in inflammatory changes of the outer gingival layers but seems unlikely to affect conditions within the gingival sulcus. This drying effect may, therefore, account for the erythematous appearance of the labial and palatal gingiva.

Periodontal Trauma

Any excessive force causing sufficient tooth displacement will produce a traumatic lesion of the supporting structures. Orthodontic forces and occlusal stress are the commonest causes of periodontal trauma. Lesions with similar pathological features will be produced by all forms of periodontal trauma. The effect of adverse occlusal forces on the periodontium is described in the next chapter, including the possible role of occlusal trauma as a modifying factor in the pathogenesis of periodontal disease.

FURTHER READING

Deasy M. J. (1980). Periodontal disease and its systemic implications. In *Efficacy of Treatment Procedures in Periodontics.* (Shanley D., ed.) p. 277. Chicago: Quintessence.

Listgarten M. A. (1987). Nature of periodontal diseases: pathogenic mechanisms. *Journal of Periodontal Research*; **22**: 172–8.

Mandel I. D., Gaffer A. (1986). Calculus revisited. A review. *Journal of Clinical Periodontology*; **13**: 249–57.

Pennel B. M., Keagle J. G. (1977). Predisposing factors in the aetiology of chronic inflammatory periodontal disease. *Journal of Periodontology*; **48**: 517–32.

Schenker B. J. (1987). Immunologic dysfunction in the pathogenesis of periodontal diseases. *Journal of Clinical Periodontology*; **14**: 489–98

Seymour R. A., Heasman P. A. (1988). Drugs and the periodontium. *Journal of Clinical Periodontology*; **15**: 1–16.

Theilade E. (1986). The non-specific theory in microbial etiology of inflammatory periodontal diseases. *Journal of Clinical Periodontology*; **13**: 905–11.

Chapter 4

Occlusal Trauma

DEFINITION

Occlusal trauma (trauma from occlusion) is an injury to any part of the masticatory system resulting from abnormal occlusal contact relationships. In the periodontal context, occlusal trauma may take two forms:

a) surface injury caused by deep overbite or food impaction;
b) injury within the connective tissue attachment apparatus as a result of excessive occlusal force transmitted by the tooth to its supporting structures. It is this form of occlusal trauma which is discussed.

ADAPTIVE PHYSIOLOGICAL RESPONSE TO OCCLUSAL FORCE

When a tooth is subjected to excessive occlusal force, it moves within its periodontium in such a way that pressure and tension zones are created in the periodontal ligament. Reorganisation within and adjacent to these zones will lead either to an increase in tooth mobility or to movement of the tooth in the direction of the applied force, or both, until the effect of the original force is nullified. During this period of adaptation, loss of definition of lamina dura may be observed on radiographs.

The mechanism for developing tooth mobility following the application of an excessive force involves an increase in periodontal ligament width, also recognisable radiographically. Adaptation is complete when the magnitude of tooth mobility or the extent of tooth migration is sufficient to accommodate or annul the displacing force. Migrated teeth will stabilise in their new position. Teeth which have maintained their position in the arch and have accommodated to the force by increasing tooth mobility will remain mobile. When adaptation is complete, new lamina dura of both migrated and hypermobile teeth may be observed radiographically, but the increased periodontal ligament space of hypermobile teeth will persist. Whether or not the

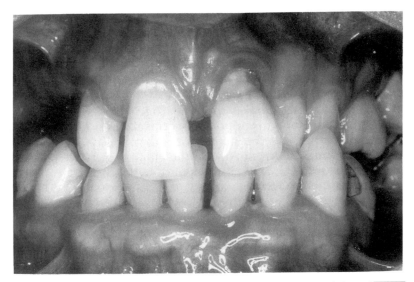

Fig. 4.1   *Occlusal disharmony and long-standing excessive mobility of 21/12.*
Oral hygiene is poor and chronic periodontitis is present.

tissue changes described above are demonstrable radiographically, will depend on how the x-ray beam angulation relates to the affected zones of the periodontium.

The development of tooth mobility or migration may, in theory, occur entirely as a physiological process if the displacing force is introduced gently, but often these tooth movements represent 'recovery phenomena' following one or more episodes of occlusal trauma.

DIAGNOSIS OF OCCLUSAL TRAUMA

The clinical diagnosis of occlusal trauma should be reserved for symptoms of periodontal pain or discomfort where the history and clinical examination support an occlusal aetiology. The traumatic lesion is characterised by a zone of increased vascularity, vascular permeability, haemorrhage and thrombosis; in severe cases, also by hyalinisation of periodontal ligament with undermining resorption of bone and cementum; and, in extreme cases, by necrosis and abscess formation.

Occlusal trauma is often transient and quickly followed by the adaptive responses outlined above, so that treatment may never be sought or required. This is probably a common sequence of events following the introduction of an inadequately contoured restoration. Except where pain is present, therefore, occlusal trauma is a diagnosis which must often be made in retrospect by the presence of tooth mobility and the radiographic appearance of a widened periodontal membrane, together with evidence of occlusal disharmony to support an occlusal aetiology (Figs. 4.1, 4.2). In this situation, the increased tooth mobility and widened periodontal membrane space are the clinical and radiographic manifestations of an adaptive response by the periodontium to accommodate the excessive forces acting on the tooth. By this time, there is probably no longer an actual traumatic lesion present, but rather a periodontal membrane which is functionally orientated to accommodate the excessive forces.

Occasionally, however, trauma may not be self-limiting, and *increasing* mobility, persistent discomfort or tenderness and

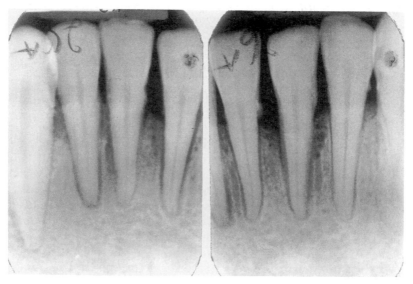

Fig. 4.2   *Radiographs of* $\overline{21/12}$ *reveal:* (a) *slight reduction in bone height with infrabony pockets typical of marginal periodontitis;* (b) *more apically, widened periodontal membrane spaces which, together with the clinical findings (see Fig. 4.1) suggest a history of occlusal trauma. There is little evidence from scientific research to support the view that occlusal trauma could have combined with marginal periodontitis to accelerate connective tissue attachment loss in this case.*

radiographic signs, such as loss of lamina dura or root resorption, point to a diagnosis of persistent occlusal trauma.

OCCLUSAL TRAUMA AS A MODIFYING FACTOR

The potential for occlusal trauma to initiate or exacerbate inflammatory periodontal disease has been the subject of much speculation for over 25 years. More recently, however, great progress has been made in our knowledge of the interactions between periodontal trauma and marginal periodontitis through a series of investigations conducted in squirrel monkeys and beagle dogs. Findings from these studies are summarised below.

a) Occlusal trauma may result in widening of the periodontal membrane, loss of crestal bone and tooth mobility, all without loss of attachment and all of which are reversible when the tooth is relieved of stress.

b) Occlusal trauma *does not* initiate or exacerbate gingivitis.

c) Occlusal trauma *does not* initiate chronic periodontitis or convert gingivitis to periodontitis.

d) Occlusal trauma *does not* initiate further loss of connective tissue attachment in a tooth with a reduced but healthy periodontium.

e) Occlusal trauma in combination with chronic periodontitis *does* result in greater tooth mobility and alveolar bone loss (but not necessarily more loss of connective tissue attachment) than either trauma or inflammation alone. Bone loss and mobility due to trauma may be reversible, but only once inflammation has been controlled, since persistent inflammation may inhibit crestal bone regeneration.

f) There is some evidence to suggest that progressive occlusal trauma in combination with marginal periodontitis *may* result in greater loss of connective tissue attachment.

g) There is *no* evidence that infrabony pockets are caused by the codestructive effect of occlusal trauma and marginal periodontitis.

Of course, pathological processes in animal models may not precisely match those in humans. Some of these conclusions, therefore, may have to be revised as more scientific knowledge becomes available.

In summary, during the last 15 years, there has been growing scepticism concerning the role of occlusal trauma in the progress of periodontal disease. Dental bacterial plaque infection has emerged as the principal target for periodontal treatment. There is mounting evidence that the progression of chronic periodontitis is episodic and it has been shown that occlusal trauma is usually transient. It seems unlikely that the notion of a codestructive effect can be sustained when one factor is episodic and the other transient.

Where progressive occlusal trauma exists, it should be treated to relieve pain or discomfort and to control increasing tooth mobility or migration. There is, however, no evidence that occlusal therapy can improve the prognosis for inflammatory periodontal disease or its treatment.

The above discussion is intended only to summarise the state of the art—refer to the recommended further reading for more information. Occlusal therapy is discussed in Chapter 15.

FURTHER READING

Ericsson I. (1986). The combined effects of plaque and physical stress on periodontal tissues. *Journal of Clinical Periodontology*; **13**: 918–22.

Polson A. M. (1986). The relative importance of plaque and occlusion in periodontal disease. *Journal of Clinical Periodontology*; **13**: 923–7.

Ramfjord S. P., Ash M. M., Jr. (1981). Significance of occlusion in the aetiology and treatment of early, moderate and advanced periodontitis. *Journal of Periodontology*; **52**: 511–17.

Waerhaug J. (1979*a*). The angular bone defect and its relationship to trauma from occlusion and subgingival plaque. *Journal of Clinical Periodontology*; **6**: 61–82.

Waerhaug J. (1979*b*). The infra bony pocket and its relationship to trauma from occlusion and subgingival plaque. *Journal of Periodontology*; **40**: 355–65.

Chapter 5

History, Examination and Diagnosis

The purpose of history taking and examination is to arrive at a diagnosis and preliminary assessment of prognosis upon which a treatment plan may be based.

Standard periodontal texts (e.g. Ramfjord and Ash, 1979) should be consulted for full details of the history taking and examination process. The purpose of this chapter is to highlight specific points, the prognostic significance of which is frequently overlooked or misunderstood.

Successful periodontal treatment makes high demands upon both patients and clinicians. It is, therefore, important that good rapport and communication be established and that efficient continuity of patient care be practised.

HISTORY

The history taking should concentrate initially on the main concerns of the patient and/or referring clinician. However, each of the common signs or symptoms of plaque-induced perio- dontal disease should be specifically inquired into. These include bleeding, pain, tooth mobility and migration, swelling, recession, bad breath and bad taste.

Bleeding

Bleeding may arise spontaneously or as a result of the mechanical stimulus of mastication or tooth cleaning. The length of history should be noted and, in particular, any sudden onset or deterioration which might suggest an underlying systemic factor.

Pain

Pain is not often a symptom of chronic gingivitis or periodontitis but is a frequent complaint and may be due to pulp disease, dentine hypersensitivity, periapical pathology, occlusal trauma or acute disease such as ulcerative gingitivis or an abscess. Frequent episodes of discomfort or pain may indicate acute disease and more rapid destruction, and should be diagnosed and treated vigorously before attempting to treat chronic, symptomless conditions.

Tooth Mobility

Patients are not always aware of increased tooth mobility. It is commonly associated with one or more of the following:

a) inflammation, marginal or apical;
b) loss of connective tissue attachment and supporting bone, usually due to marginal periodontal disease but occasionally due to periapical disease;
c) increase in width of periodontal membrane, usually due to occlusal forces.

Patients who complain of or are aware of mobility should be asked about its duration and whether it appears to have increased since first noted. Any masticatory difficulty due to mobility such as discomfort or food impaction should also be noted.

While mobility may be a sign of disease, it may also be a sign of physiological adaptation to reduced support or increased function, and should by no means be invariably interpreted as a sign of poor prognosis or indication for extraction. Patients may need to be reassured about this. However, *increasing* mobility may indicate rapid loss of support and should receive urgent attention if tooth loss is to be avoided.

Some decrease in mobility may follow control of inflammation, occlusal adjustment and periodontal surgery (after a temporary increase in mobility). Although splinting may lead to some decrease in mobility, following removal of the splint, mobility will return gradually to previous levels. Decrease in mobility may be taken as a favourable prognostic indicator. However, when periodontal support is reduced, some mobility must be expected to persist in spite of thorough treatment including occlusal adjustment. If tooth mobility interferes with comfort or function, or seems to be increasing, splinting may be indicated.

Tooth Migration

Patients are usually aware of migration of anterior teeth because of the development of spaces. Again the duration of such changes should be noted. Old photographs may occasionally be useful. Migration may take place even when the periodontium is healthy, although it is more likely when there has been loss of support. It reflects the disruption of the normal balance of forces acting on teeth and supporting bone. Migration may, therefore, be due to loss of an adjacent tooth, occlusal stress or activity of the oral musculature, and usually affects teeth with poor crown:root ratios. It may occur without significant mobility. If orthodontic correction is possible, permanent retention will frequently be required. Migration may occur spontaneously or as a result of parafunctional habits. Elimination of habits may occasionally allow spontaneous realignment without appliance therapy.

The players of certain musical wind instruments with intraoral mouthpieces or reeds may suffer tooth migration due to periodontal disease and the parafunctional presence of the mouthpiece. Playing will have adapted as the teeth gradually migrate and difficulty may be experienced if an attempt is made to realign the natural teeth or replace them with a prosthesis.

MEDICAL HISTORY

A careful medical history must be taken from all patients and periodically updated. The objectives are:

a)   to note the existence of systemic factors which may have helped to account for the periodontal condition, i.e. pregnancy, diabetes mellitus, etc. (Chapter 3);

b)   to note the existence of systemic factors for which special precautions will be necessary to safeguard the patient during periodontal therapy, e.g. patients with valvular disorders of the heart will require antibiotic cover to reduce the risk of infective endocarditis following periodontal instrumentation;

c)   to alert the clinician to any disease processes which present a hazard to himself, his staff or other patients, e.g. cross-infection may occur from patients with a history of viral hepatitis B.

EXAMINATION

Examination should reveal the extent and severity of the disease with a view to advising the patient of the treatment options and the likely prognosis.

A systematic examination should lead to a full diagnosis including the diseases or conditions present and their extent and severity, e.g. whether localised or generalised, early or advanced.

Gingival Inflammation, Microbial Plaque and Calculus

Gingivitis may be recognised by the characteristic appearance of inflammation, such as change of colour from pink to red and enlargement due to oedema or hyperplasia (*see* Fig. 2.2). Gingival exudate may be evident if the teeth are first dried. Bleeding will usually occur when a periodontal probe is run along the soft-tissue wall at the entrance to the gingival pocket. Suppuration and ulceration may indicate acute inflammation, such as an abscess or ulcerative gingivitis.

Plaque or calculus deposits will invariably be found in contact with the inflamed tissue and, generally, the severity of inflammation will correlate with the amount of plaque. Typically, little plaque will be found on buccal tooth surfaces but it will be evident on the lingual aspects of lower posterior teeth which are less accessible, and the proximal surfaces which are inadequately cleaned with a toothbrush. Other combinations of clean and plaque-infected surfaces should be noted and the explanation sought.

There is a great variation between individuals in the tendency for mineralisation of plaque. Supragingival calculus is easy to remove, and once excellent plaque control is established there are few individuals in whom supragingival calculus will continue to form. The amount of subgingival calculus is also subject to considerable variation between individuals. It is extremely adherent and its presence in large amounts points to a prolonged phase of hygiene therapy.

The progress of hygiene therapy may be monitored by means of indices. Many indices are complex and time consuming to employ and are, therefore, unsuitable for clinical practice. The O'Leary plaque index (O'Leary *et al.*, 1972) is recommended. This simply records the presence or absence of plaque in contact with the gingival margin of selected sites. The gingival bleeding index (Ainamo and Bay, 1975) records the presence or absence of bleeding from the gingival margin, elicited by a periodontal probe. These indices are only suitable when the objective of treatment is regarded as perfect plaque control and total gingival health, as they do not incorporate a severity scale, which is sacrificed for simplicity.

An index of gingival health is generally more informative than an index of plaque. Some patients may achieve very low plaque indices but may do so only to impress the dentist at the time of appointment. Such patients will not achieve significant improvement of their gingival inflammation index. Furthermore, gingivitis may persist in the absence of supragingival plaque, due to the presence of subgingival deposits.

Finally, one must be wary of forming an impression of attachment levels purely on the amount of plaque and calculus and the severity of gingival inflammation. Severe gingivitis may be present without attachment loss, or attachment loss may be present without gingivitis if supragingival plaque control has improved since the onset of periodontitis.

Periodontal Probing

The periodontal probe can be used to assess pocket depths and to identify pockets which bleed on probing.

Pocket depths. The depth to which the periodontal probe will penetrate beyond the gingival margin depends on:

a)   the amount of gingival enlargement;
b)   the extent of connective tissue attachment loss;
c)   the resistance of the tissue to probing, determined by the integrity of the epithelial barrier and the extent to which gingival collagen has been replaced by inflammatory infiltrate;
d)   size, shape and tip diameter of the probe;
e)   use of the probe—pressure applied and angle of insertion (this has been found to vary widely between and within operators);
f)   the presence of obstructions such as subgingival calculus;
g)   the patient's reaction to the discomfort of probing.

These factors illustrate why the true depth of the pocket may not be accurately recorded by probing and the expression 'probing depth' is now often used instead of the more traditional 'pocket depth' when referring to the results of an examination with the periodontal probe. The probing (or pocket) depth, nevertheless, may give the best indication of the severity and extent of periodontal disease compared with other clinical or radiographic parameters. Furthermore, the probing depth gives a rough indication of the likely response to treatment. That is because adequate débridement becomes more difficult as probing depths increase. Within the range 3–5 mm, adequate subgingival scaling and root planing is unpredictable and pockets of 5 mm or more frequently require surgical intervention.

The probing distance from the amelocemental junction to the base of the pocket gives the amount of attachment loss. However, in determining the ultimate prognosis of the tooth, proper consideration must be given to the amount of *residual* supporting tissue, which may be gauged to some extent by mobility tests and by reference to radiographs.

Bleeding. The cardinal sign of a pathological pocket is bleeding on probing, as the instrument breaches the ulcerated and inflamed pocket wall. In patients with untreated periodontal disease, generally, all pockets of around 3 mm and over will bleed on probing. On the other hand, where a long junctional epithelium has formed, consequent upon successful treatment, probing depths may exceed 3 mm without eliciting a bleeding response from this healthy but penetrable epithelium. Whereas it is generally accepted that bleeding on probing is the cardinal sign of disease, there is no evidence that the amount of bleeding is related to the rate of attachment loss or to the likelihood of further loss of attachment. The reader is referred to the review article by Listgarten (1980) for a detailed appraisal of periodontal probing. Setchell and Shaw (1980) describe the physical characteristics of different periodontal probes.

Occlusion, Mobility and Migration

The emphasis in examination of occlusion should be on features which might exacerbate disease or make successful treatment difficult or impossible. Thus, features which complicate plaque control or lead to trauma or food impaction should be noted. If mobility is present the occlusion should be checked for premature or interfering contacts and for evidence of food impaction. Various systems exist to classify mobility. Most are based on subjective judgements. One system is recommended in

Appendix I. Mobility can be related crudely to the extent and severity of chronic periodontitis. Where tooth mobility appears to be disproportionately large in relation to other clinical signs of disease there may be evidence of occlusal stress and occlusal therapy may be indicated (*see* Chapter 15). If possible, a final decision on occlusal therapy should be delayed until the response to hygiene therapy can be observed. It should be remembered that a temporary increase in mobility frequently takes place after surgery and temporary splinting may help to limit this as well as facilitate scaling and root planing during surgery. Mobility in teeth with furcation lesions is usually a late sign and generally indicates a poor prognosis. Such teeth are unlikely to be candidates for root separation techniques, as a further increase in mobility can be anticipated once the 'tripod' or 'bipod' of roots is divided.

Among the many forms of tooth migration, anterior tooth migration is the most unacceptable because of the effect on aesthetics. The case history should have established whether any parafunctional habits may have been responsible. The occlusion should now be examined as a potential contributory factor (*see* Chapter 15). Unfortunately, upper anterior tooth migration is often accompanied by over-eruption of the affected tooth and of its antagonist in the lower arch. Such changes complicate orthodontic treatment.

Mucogingival Relationships

The terms 'attached' and 'keratinised' gingiva should be distinguished. Keratinised gingiva is only 'attached' where periosteal or dentogingival attachment exists coronal to the mucogingival line. Thus, marginal bone loss will lead to loss of attached gingiva but not to loss of keratinised gingiva unless there is also recession.

Where plaque and gingivitis are present on buccal or lingual surfaces, mucogingival relationships should be assessed. For example, a shallow vestibule or a high fraenum attachment may impair access for adequate plaque control, while a lack of keratinised gingiva may result in mucosal trauma during tooth brushing. Provided access exists for adequate and atraumatic plaque control, the actual gingival width, according to recent research, is unimportant, a narrow band of gingiva being no more susceptible to inflammation should plaque be allowed to accumulate.

Lip-pull tests, to demonstrate blanching or movement of the gingival margin, have been used to assess the need for mucogingival surgery. Manipulation of lip and cheek in this way, however, is not physiological and such tests are, therefore, meaningless.

Chapter 13 is devoted to the aetiology and management of mucogingival problems.

Furcation Lesions

The frequency and extent of furcation lesions are usually underestimated and this may be due to inadequate assessment of root anatomy, reliance on the straight periodontal probe rather than exploration with a curved instrument such as a curette and to misinterpretation of radiographs which almost invariably do not reveal the true extent of involvement. Furcations should be checked carefully so that the feasibility of satisfactory treatment can be assessed. It should be remembered that proximal furcation lesions may affect the support of adjacent teeth unless they are separated by a particularly broad inter-radicular septum.

Generally, the mesial furcation of upper molars is more easily examined from the palatal side, the distal furcation from the buccal. This is because the mesiobuccal root is broader buccopalatally than the distobuccal root and the palatal root is situated distopalatally (*see* Fig. 11.1).

Radiographs

Radiographs cannot be used to diagnose current periodontal disease since they cannot show whether marginal bone loss is associated with inflamed tissues or with tissues which have been restored to health as a result of successful treatment.

Radiographs are, however, necessary to assess the proportion of support lost in relation to root length. Periapical radiographs, taken with the 'long cone paralleling' technique, are most useful. Inevitably, however, there are limitations to the use of radiographs in periodontics because of the superimposition of tooth on bone and cortical bone on cancellous bone. Thus, buccal and/or lingual bone margins may be visible inter-proximally but interdental infrabony defects, including furcation lesions, may be wholly or partially obscured.

The appearance of the crestal bone is a function of x-ray beam angulation and cannot be relied upon as an indicator of disease activity or healing. Indeed, there are no radiographic features which indicate whether disease is progressing or static. It should be remembered that, although a gingival soft-tissue shadow may be visible, radiographs do not reveal pockets.

Radiographs will also reveal unerupted teeth, periapical pathology, inadequate endodontic treatment, caries, overhanging margins, etc., which may have a bearing on tooth prognosis or the planning of subsequent restorative treatment. It may be reasonable, for example, to combine apicectomy with a periodontal flap procedure.

Special techniques such as 'parallax' may occasionally be useful, as may the use of gutta-percha or metal points to indicate pocket depth or periodontal–apical communication.

The reader is referred to the review article by Lang and Hill (1977) for further details.

Study Casts

Assessment of occlusal relationships will often be facilitated by mounted study casts.

Special Tests

Pulp vitality tests should be carried out for teeth associated with deep periodontal pockets where pulpitis or pulp necrosis may have resulted from periodontal disease. Vitality tests may also help to distinguish a periapical from a periodontal abscess. In this respect, multirooted teeth require careful interpretation (*see* Chapter 12).

Haematological investigations such as a full blood count and film are indicated where blood dyscrasias such as neutropenia, leukaemia or thrombocytopenia are suspected.

DIAGNOSIS

A classification of periodontal disease is given in Appendix III. It is usually possible to make a diagnosis which describes the predominant feature, e.g. chronic gingivitis or chronic periodontitis. This, however, is not particularly informative as most adults have teeth which are affected by chronic gingivitis as well as teeth affected by chronic periodontitis. Different teeth or even different gingival sites of individual teeth may show variations from absolute health to advanced destructive disease. Ideally, therefore, a tooth-by-tooth diagnosis should be made at the patient's initial examination and again following hygiene therapy.

Patients presenting with symptoms of periodontal disease will require a thorough examination before treatment, and numerous systems exist for recording the results of detailed examination procedures. The example illustrated in Appendix I has space reserved for recording probing depth measurements for each tooth surface, tooth mobility scores and furcation lesions. The treatment required can be individually determined for each tooth. A detailed assessment of this type is desirable at the patient's first visit and essential after hygiene therapy to determine the need, if any, for more elaborate treatment procedures.

For a simple and rapid method of recording periodontal conditions during a routine dental examination, the reader is referred to Appendix II, where a technique is described for estimating periodontal treatment needs, based on the Community Periodontal Index of Treatment Needs (CPITN). A severity code is given to each 'sextant' indicating roughly the complexity of treatment likely to be required.

This system has been devised by the British Society of Periodontology for use in general dental practice in the United Kingdom. Its main virtue, when compared with tooth-by-tooth charting and diagnosis, is its suitability for 'screening' all patients in general dental practice for periodontal disease. Screening can be carried out more quickly than a full periodontal assessment, which would be inappropriate for most patients attending for routine dental examination. It cannot, however, replace full periodontal assessment in patients with significant periodontal problems. Comprehensive examination will, therefore, be required to select hopeless teeth for extraction, to establish the extent of furcation lesions, to diagnose combined periodontal–endodontic lesions and to evaluate the full extent and significance of mucogingival problems.

REFERENCES

Ainamo J., Bay I. (1975). Problems and proposals for recording gingivitis and plaque. *International Dental Journal*; **25**: 229–35.

Lang N. P., Hill R. W. (1977). Radiographs in periodontics. *Journal of Clinical Periodontology*; **4**: 16–28.

Listgarten M. (1980). Periodontal probing: What does it mean? *Journal of Clinical Periodontology*; **7**: 165–76.

O'Leary T. J., Drake R. B., Naylor J. E. (1972). The plaque control record. *Journal of Periodontology*; **43**: 38.

Ramfjord S. P., Ash M. M., Jr. (1979). Examination and diagnosis. In *Periodontology and Periodontics*. Ch. 11. Eastbourne: W. B. Saunders.

Setchell D. J., Shaw M. J. (1980). The graduated periodontal probe. *Dental Update*; **7**: 431–9.

FURTHER READING

Ainamo J., Barnes D., Beagrie G., Cutress T., Martin J., Sardo-Infirri J. (1982). Development of the World Health Organization (WHO) Community Periodontal Index of Treatment Needs (CPITN). *International Dental Journal*; **32**: 281–91.

Chapter 6

Rationale of Treatment

EPIDEMIOLOGY AND TREATMENT NEED

It is well established that periodontal disease is extremely common, being more prevalent and more severe with rising age and in individuals with poor oral hygiene. Furthermore, in primitive regions where oral hygiene is neglected, periodontal disease experience is greater than in developed countries where ritual, if not entirely effective, toothbrushing is practised.

Owing to a lack of universally acceptable diagnostic criteria, epidemiological surveys, even of similar populations, have produced conflicting data on the amount of periodontal disease. The figures discussed below apply only to developed countries and are in most cases tentative.

Gingivitis is present in most mouths. Periodontitis is rarely observed before puberty and usually commences in adolescence or early adulthood. It is reported to affect between about 1–50% of adolescents and about 50–100% of middle-aged adults, the prevalence rising with increasing age. Also with increasing age, a greater number of teeth become involved and there is an increasing severity of attachment loss. The mean rate of periodontal destruction is believed to be about 0·1–0·2 mm of connective tissue attachment per year, but it varies considerably between individuals and between individual tooth surfaces and may amount to several millimetres over a period of a few months at certain sites during an active phase of the disease.

It is thought that approximately 90% of individuals with periodontitis suffer from *simple* periodontitis, which progresses at a relatively slow rate, consistent usually with lifetime tooth survival. The remaining 10% suffer, during at least one stage in their life, from *complex* periodontitis, where there is a gross imbalance of host–parasite equilibrium resulting in rapidly progressive destruction around one or more teeth in adolescence (juvenile periodontitis) or adulthood (*see* Appendix III).

It is generally agreed that, over the age of 35 to 40 years, more *teeth* are lost through periodontitis than through caries;

however, fewer *individuals* lose teeth through periodontitis. This is because advanced periodontitis affects a large number of teeth in a comparatively small proportion of the population. Schaub (1984) has estimated that tooth loss due to periodontitis affects only 10–15% of the adult dentate population but causes approximately half of this group to lose most of their teeth.

PROGNOSIS

Longitudinal studies (e.g. Becker *et al.*, 1979) have confirmed that untreated periodontal disease leads to continued loss of support, increased pocket depth and eventual tooth loss. On the other hand, numerous clinical trials and retrospective studies (for review, see Kakehashi and Parakkal, 1982) have documented the effectiveness of various forms of treatment in controlling periodontal disease. Reporting on the long-term maintenance of 61 patients treated for advanced periodontal disease, Lindhe and Nyman (1984) found that only 0·1% of sites per year showed evidence of further attachment loss. Two groups of untreated subjects, by comparison, experienced attachment loss at 1·9% and 3·2% of sites per year. Thus proper periodontal treatment and maintenance care may reduce the frequency of sites with disease progression by a factor of 20 to 30 times.

TIME REQUIRED FOR TREATMENT

Several studies have attempted to quantify the time required for periodontal treatment. One such study (Johansen *et al* ., 1973) calculated the time spent in periodontal treatment for a group of 42 patients. The average time spent in motivation and instruction during the course of treatment amounted to 1 hour 12 minutes per patient. Scaling took 5 minutes per tooth and surgery took 11 minutes per tooth.

Obviously, the time required for treatment will depend on the extent of the disease and on the objective of treatment. Hill *et al.* (1981) reported that preoperative scaling and oral hygiene instruction for a group of 90 patients with moderate to severe chronic periodontitis required between five and eight hours per individual over four or five appointments. Following resolution of periodontal disease, maintenance care is required at approximately three-monthly intervals indefinitely.

In considering the large treatment need and the time required for treatment, it is obvious that treatment leading to periodontal health cannot be pursued indiscriminately or indefinitely. Each practitioner must, therefore, consider what his objective should be in the light of his patient's response to initial treatment procedures.

OBJECTIVES OF TREATMENT

Relief of Symptoms

Although in many cases complete restoration of periodontal health is unattainable, the relief of symptoms, which in turn leads to a sense of personal well-being, is an important objective for the clinician. 'Success' in periodontal therapy should not be measured only by the yardstick of restored periodontal health.

Provision of Optimum Conditions for Self-performed Plaque Control

Dental health education and oral hygiene instruction are key items in all aspects of periodontal treatment, but so too is the elimination of factors whose presence inhibits adequate self-performed plaque control. These factors include calculus, malpositioned or badly restored teeth and unfavourable gingival contours or mucogingival relationships.

Restoration and Maintenance of Function and Aesthetics

Diminished chewing function may result from excessive tooth mobility or tooth migration. A migrated anterior tooth may also be unaesthetic. Treatment cannot be considered complete until such teeth are restored to function and stabilised within the arch. Occasionally, gross gingival hyperplasia may be present, and, as well as being unaesthetic, the gingival surface may be traumatised by the opposing teeth. In such cases, periodontal treatment should include measures to restore function and aesthetics.

Restoration of Periodontal Health

Periodontal health can be defined as absence of both inflammation and progressive breakdown of the gingiva and supporting tissues of the tooth. At the dentogingival junction, there will be a *physiological gingival sulcus* recognisable clinically by the absence of bleeding on probing.

From a public health standpoint, this must be regarded as an idealistic goal. A more realistic public health objective is an improved standard of periodontal health and thereby a reduction in the rate of attachment loss to a level compatible with tooth survival. The amount and type of care to achieve this reduced goal is, however, indefinable since the potential for periodontal breakdown varies greatly between individuals and between different teeth in the same mouth; at present there are no known 'prognostic indicators' which would allow the most susceptible patients and teeth to be singled out for priority treatment. Furthermore, there are many individuals for whom the mere survival of teeth is unacceptable unless the periodontal tissue will exist in a state of health.

Somewhere, a balance must be struck between the patient's subjective needs, the clinician's therapeutic objectives and the available resources. The answer is to plan periodontal treatment in a stepwise progression: if elaborate treatment procedures are required which are dependent on good oral hygiene, these are deferred until initial progress has been assessed; patients who maintain a positive attitude will, thereby, achieve the highest standards of periodontal health.

The best available follow-up approach to patients who make a poor response to initial therapy is a programme of professional tooth cleaning at frequent intervals. However, to be fully effective this must be implemented thoughtfully, since it is unlikely that complete tooth débridement will be achieved in one recall visit for patients with widespread periodontal disease. The clinician will have to decide which teeth are of greatest strategic importance so that the major treatment effort may be concentrated at sites where treatment is most required, instead of being dissipated throughout the dentition. At the present time, in the absence of a reliable index of disease activity, this may represent the best approach to the treatment of patients whose standards of home care are not consistent with periodontal health. Such patients form the majority of the dentate population.

The ground rules for treatment leading to absolute periodontal health are much simpler than those which govern palliative treatment. Since the criteria of periodontal health are well defined and readily identifiable, the end-point of treatment is easily recognised. The comments on treatment in the remainder of this chapter are made with the assumption that the objective of treatment is complete periodontal health—a physiological gingival sulcus.

STRUCTURAL CHANGES AFTER TREATMENT

The formation of a physiological sulcus is a feature common to the healing of all inflammatory periodontal lesions, but the structural organisation of the underlying connective tissues will depend on the damage previously inflicted.

Treatment of Gingivitis

Figure 6.1 illustrates a limited gingivitis (Fig 6.1(a)) and the structure of the gingiva (Fig 6.1(b)) once healing has taken place following removal of plaque and calculus. The pocket epithelium undergoes transition to junctional epithelium which forms an attachment to the adjacent tooth surface. The inflammatory

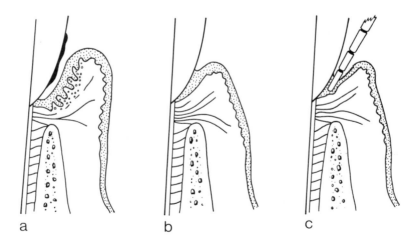

a   b   c

Fig. 6.1   *Treatment of gingivitis. (a) Gingivitis. (b) Normal healthy periodontium after treatment. (c) 'Normal' probing depth after treatment.*

infiltrate is gradually replaced by maturing collagen fibres which eventually become organised into functionally orientated bundles. Clinically these healing events are manifested as a change to a uniform pink colour, a reduction in gingival bulk and the formation of a physiological gingival sulcus with a 'normal' probing depth of 1–2 mm (Fig. 6.1(c)). Gingivitis then, from both a clinical and histological viewpoint, is reversible. Tissues are restored not just to health but also to normality. This may necessitate surgical excision if gross fibrous enlargement has occurred.

Treatment of Periodontitis

Periodontitis is characterised by loss of connective tissue attachment (Fig. 6.2(a) and Fig. 6.3(a)). Successful treatment depends on the removal of plaque, calculus and contaminated cementum accompanied by very good plaque control. This leads to elimination of inflammation with *repair* but not *regeneration* of the supporting tissues. Similar results may be achieved with or without surgical access. Following subgingival scaling and root planing, remnants of pocket epithelium will be transformed into junctional epithelium which will cover the tooth surface down to

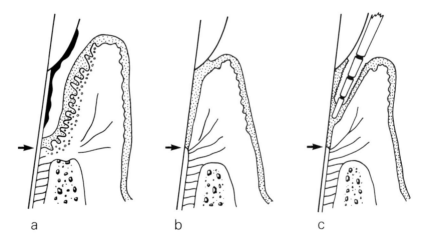

a   b   c

Fig. 6.2   *Treatment of periodontitis (suprabony pocket): arrows indicate connective tissue attachment levels.* (a) *Periodontitis with suprabony pocket.* (b) *Reduced healthy periodontium after treatment.* (c) *Gain in clinical attachment after treatment.*

the base of the original pocket (Fig. 6.2(b) and Fig. 6.3(b)). Even if the pocket lining is surgically excised, such is the rapidity of epithelial cell migration that the entire area of denuded root becomes covered with junctional epithelium before other tissue cells in the vicinity have colonised any part of the exposed root. The junctional epithelium forms a long epithelial attachment. In the underlying connective tissues, the inflammatory infiltrate will be replaced by collagen but the junctional epithelium will, of course, form a barrier to new fibre attachment.

In the case of a suprabony pocket, the supporting bone will undergo very little change, although after surgery there might be a slight loss of crestal bone height.

Some infrabony pockets, particularly those with three bone walls, may exhibit bone-fill (Fig. 6.3(b)), although surgical curettage of the defect may be necessary to initiate bone regeneration, and this is likely to cause a slight loss of crestal bone height. It should be noted that bone-fill of infrabony pockets is not accompanied by new connective tissue attachment. Instead, the underlying root surface will be lined with junctional epithelium (Fig. 6.3(b)).

The structural changes described above involve healing with a long junctional epithelium. An alternative approach to the

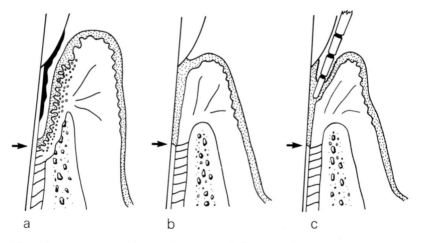

a   b   c

Fig. 6.3 *Treatment of periodontitis (infrabony pocket): arrows represent connective tissue attachment levels. (a) Periodontitis with infrabony pocket. (b) Reduced healthy periodontium with bone-fill after treatment. (c) Gain in clinical attachment after treatment.*

treatment of periodontitis uses surgery not just to gain access to root surface deposits but also to 'eliminate' the soft-tissue and hard-tissue pocket walls to produce a dentogingival attachment of normal dimensions and with a limited epithelial component. This approach is based on the assumption that the barrier function of a long junctional epithelium against plaque infection may be inferior to that of a normal dentogingival attachment. Limited evidence to date, however, has failed to show any appreciable difference in resistance to disease between a long epithelial attachment and a true connective tissue attachment following a period of unsatisfactory plaque control (Magnusson *et al.*, 1983; Beaumont *et al.*, 1984).

Clinically, following successful treatment of periodontitis, the gingiva should appear uniformly pink and firm, and some gingival recession will inevitably have occurred, more so after surgery. Tooth mobility may have decreased. Most significantly, with the formation of a physiological gingival sulcus, there should be no bleeding on probing. There will be a reduction in probing depths, although, because of the absence of bone close to the gingival margin and the friability of the junctional epithelium, it may be possible to record pocket depths which are greater than 'normal'. The magnitude of the reduction in clinical pocket depth depends on the extent of gingival recession and the gain in clinical attachment, if any.

Attachment Gain

Figures 6.2 and 6.3 show that treatment of periodontitis does not result in an improvement in connective tissue attachment level (arrowed). The connective tissue attachment level, that is the point on the root to which the most coronal fibres are attached, can be precisely identified only by histology. However, in the presence of periodontitis, it corresponds roughly to the base of the pocket and so can be identified by probing. After healing, however, because of the improved gingival tone and bone-fill, if any, penetration of the probe will be reduced, giving an apparent gain in attachment. The magnitude of this clinical attachment gain in Figures 6.2(c) and 6.3(c) corresponds to the distance between the arrow (formerly the base of the pocket) and the probe tip. As a general rule, the deeper the pocket, the greater the gain in clinical attachment. The resistance to probing after treatment may mask an underlying true loss of attachment due to instrumentation trauma.

TREATMENT MODALITIES

Dental Health Education and Instruction

Plaque forms continuously and the objective of oral hygiene instruction is to advise the patient how plaque may be successfully removed with a frequency sufficient to prevent pathological effects arising from recurrent plaque accumulation. Motivation is an essential factor in establishing a pattern of behaviour which will make the patient independent of professional support. Chemical antiplaque agents are available to augment mechanical methods, but none are without side-effects. Chlorhexidine, for example, stains teeth and fillings and causes disturbances of taste.

Scaling and Root Planing

The achievement of satisfactory levels of plaque control in a healthy mouth should be sufficient to prevent the onset of gingivitis and the subsequent development of periodontitis. If inflammation is allowed to occur, however, it will be accompanied by the establishment of a subgingival pocket flora which, except at the entrance of the sulcus, will survive personal oral hygiene measures and maintain the inflammatory process. Subgingival débridement is, therefore, of fundamental importance in pocket therapy. Where pockets are shallow, subgingival instrumentation may suffice to eliminate all toxic substances and allow repair to occur with the formation of a physiological gingival sulcus. The deeper the pocket, however, the less effective will this treatment be and the greater the need for surgical intervention.

Nevertheless, it must not be assumed that surgery is unavoidable for the successful management of advanced periodontal disease. In recent years, a number of reports, reviewed by Pihlstrom *et al.* (1983), have emerged showing that, in the treatment of deep pockets, periodontal health can be established by prolonged and meticulous scaling and root planing without the need for surgery. Indeed, according to Lindhe *et al.* (1982), significantly more gain in clinical attachment is achieved by the modified Widman flap approach (*see* Chapter 10) than by prolonged scaling and root planing only when pocket depths exceed 7 mm. These results, however, were achieved under experimental conditions and only after an extended period of instrumentation and may not, therefore, be readily reproducible in routine clinical practice. Subgingival scaling, furthermore, unless carried out with local anaesthetic, is an unpleasant experience for most patients as the instrument is in constant contact with sensitive periodontal and dental tissue.

A further practical difficulty exists when subgingival scaling and root planing are considered as definitive treatment for advanced periodontal disease. Where a large number of deep pathological pockets exists throughout the mouth, it is improbable that all will respond, even to prolonged scaling and root planing procedures. In spite of many visits for non-surgical débridement, therefore, surgical intervention may still be necessary for one or two teeth, perhaps in each quadrant, prolonging the treatment time further. In the final analysis, the prospect of achieving complete removal of root surface irritants from deep pockets without surgical access will be determined by the clinician's skill and experience.

Accordingly, the approach to pocket therapy, recommended in this text and discussed in more detail in Chapters 7, 9, and 10, is briefly explained thus: treatment should commence with a phase of hygiene therapy (motivation, instruction, scaling and root planing) which should proceed until the patient reaches his peak level of plaque control and all reasonably accessible subgingival deposits have been removed; at this point the patient is re-examined and, if pathological pockets, i.e. pockets which bleed or exude pus on probing, persist at sites of near-perfect plaque control, surgical intervention should be considered.

We would venture to suggest that in routine clinical practice pockets of 3 mm or less should always be amenable to treatment by non-surgical débridement; for pockets of about 3–5 mm, complete non-surgical débridement should always be attempted but may not always be successful. Without surgical intervention, pockets in excess of 5 mm will often persist. The studies of Waerhaug (1978) on extracted teeth lend support to this approach.

Experienced clinicians may be able to predict at the patient's initial visit which jaw segments can be treated adequately by a non-surgical approach and which segments are likely to require surgical intervention. In the latter case, subgingival instrumentation may be curtailed once the gross subgingival deposits have been removed. Subject to the establishment of good plaque control, treatment may then be completed surgically without delay, sparing the patient a protracted phase of non-surgical root instrumentation with little expectation of success. Of course, even when surgical intervention appears unavoidable, gross subgingival deposits must first be removed. This will reduce the level of inflammation and improve tissue consistency, thereby permitting improved visibility and better tissue handling during surgery.

In recent years new treatment strategies involving topical and systemic chemotherapy have been suggested in the management of chronic periodontitis. Since these remain at the experimental stage they are discussed in Chapter 20.

Surgical Treatment

Surgical treatment may occasionally be required to excise grossly hyperplastic gingiva or to improve mucogingival relationships, to facilitate improved self-performed plaque control. Severe gingival hyperplasia may also require surgical intervention for cosmetic reasons. The principal use of surgery, however, is in the treatment of advanced periodontitis (surgical pocket therapy) where the foremost objective is the provision of access for more effective root instrumentation. Whatever technique of surgical pocket therapy is chosen, it is essential that satisfactory gingival contours are produced and it may, therefore, be necessary to remove bone and excise or apically reposition the soft tissue. Wherever possible, the full potential for repair should be exploited by preserving bone and replacing soft tissue to give the results depicted in Figures 6.2(b) and 6.3(b).

It is apparent that surgical pocket therapy is reserved for patients with comparatively advanced disease, that is, for patients who have shown the greatest susceptibility to plaque infection. It is, therefore, not surprising that a large number of carefully controlled clinical studies have demonstrated a high rate of recurrence where surgery was not supported by a very high standard of personal plaque control. These reports lead to the conclusion that however deep the pocket, whatever verbal reassurance with respect to oral hygiene is given by the patient, however anxious he or she may be to conclude treatment, surgery should *not* be attempted without visible evidence of near-perfect plaque control at the reassessment stage following hygiene therapy. The patient must also understand that this level of plaque control will need to be maintained by effective home care and regular professional cleaning.

MAINTENANCE CARE

A phase of maintenance care should follow the conclusion of active treatment regardless of whether surgery has been carried out.

At the completion of therapy it should be possible for the patient to have access to all sites at which plaque will form. Nevertheless, reinforcement of oral hygiene instruction at frequent intervals is essential. Furthermore, supragingival calculus deposits may continue to form and must be removed. The subject of recall maintenance is discussed in greater detail in Chapter 16.

REFERENCES

Beaumont R. H., O'Leary T. J., Kafrawy A. H. (1984). Relative resistance of long junctional epithelial adhesions and connective tissue attachments to plaque-induced inflammation. *Journal of Periodontology*; **55**: 213–23.

Becker W., Berg L., Becker B. E. (1979). Untreated periodontal disease: a longitudinal study. *Journal of Periodontology*; **50**: 234–44.

Hill R. W., Ramfjord S. P., Morrison E. C., *et al.* (1981). Four types of periodontal treatment compared over two years. *Journal of Periodontology*; **52**: 655–62.

Johansen J. R., Gjermo F., Bellini H. T. (1973). A system to classify the need for periodontal treatment. *Acta Odontologica Scandinavica*; **31**: 297–305.

Kakehashi S., Parakkal P. F. (1982). Surgical therapy for periodontitis. *Journal of Periodontology*; **53**: 475–501.

Lindhe J., Socransky S. S., Nyman S., Haffajee A., Westfeldt E. (1982). 'Critical probing depths' in periodontal therapy. *Journal of Clinical Periodontology*; **9**: 323–36.

Lindhe J., Nyman S. (1984). Long-term maintenance of patients treated for advanced periodontal disease. *Journal of Clinical Periodontology*; **11**: 504–14.

Magnusson I., Runstad L., Nyman S., Lindhe J. (1983). A long junctional epithelium—a locus minoris resistentiae in plaque infection? *Journal of Clinical Periodontology*; **10**: 333–40.

Pihlstrom B. L., McHugh R. B., Oliphant T. H., Ortiz-Campos C. (1983). Comparison of surgical and non surgical treatment of periodontal disease. A review of current studies and additional results after 6½ years. *Journal of Clinical Periodontology*; **10**: 524–41.

Schaub R. M. H. (1984). *Barriers to Effective Periodontal Care.* Thesis, University of Groningen.

Waerhaug J. (1978). Healing of the dento-epithelial junction following sub-gingival plaque control. II As observed on extracted teeth. *Journal of Periodontology*; **49**: 119–34.

FURTHER READING

Loe, H., Anerud A., Boysen H., Morrison E. (1986). Natural history of periodontal disease in man. Rapid, moderate and no loss of attachment in Sri Lankan laborers 14 to 46 years of age. *Journal of Clinical Periodontology*; **13**: 431–40.

Page R. C., Schroeder H. E. (1982). Periodontitis in humans. In *Periodontitis in Man and Other Animals.* pp. 5–17. Basle: Karger.

Pilot T. (1986). Economic perspectives on diagnosis and treatment planning in periodontology. *Journal of Clinical Periodontology*; **13**: 889–94.

Stamm J. W. (1986). Epidemiology of gingivitis. *Journal of Clinical Periodontology*; **13**: 360–6.

Chapter 7

Treatment Planning

Treatment planning is the process by which significance is attached to clinical findings and decisions are made about the action to be taken.

The *general aim* should be to satisfy the patient's functional and aesthetic requirements within the limits of available resources of expertise, time and technique, with a reasonable prognosis. This will sometimes entail a degree of compromise.

RATIONALE OF TREATMENT PLANNING

The main aetiological agent in periodontal disease is microbial plaque. The severity and rate of progression of disease depend on the nature of the plaque and on its interactions with the host. Since the means by which plaque causes loss of connective tissue attachment and the nature of the host response are not fully understood, the main emphasis in treatment must be on elimination of plaque. Effective plaque control will also reduce caries.

Periodontal treatment cannot be divorced from other restorative procedures, and so an overall treatment for the patient must be planned. Study casts and radiographs are invaluable to supplement clinical examination, to facilitate discussion with the patient and as pretreatment records.

During treatment planning, it is necessary to recognise that wide variation exists in severity of disease in relation to oral hygiene and age. Patients also differ in motivation, manual dexterity and availability for treatment. These factors must be taken into account, albeit somewhat subjectively, so that the aims of the operator and expectations of the patient are correlated as closely as possible before treatment begins. The role of the dentist is advisory as well as technical and, while one should not try to *persuade* patients to have treatment, they should be directed to an appropriate course of action, and then allowed to decide what priority they wish to give their oral health. Faced with the prospect of losing teeth through periodontal disease, most patients will opt for treatment. Few, however, have the remotest concept of the nature and duration of treatment and the personal commitment required to achieve periodontal health. It is the clinician's duty to make patients fully aware of the time and effort required.

PHASES OF TREATMENT

The following sequence should not be seen as inflexible.

a) Relief of acute symptoms (*see* Chapter 18).
b) i) Hygiene therapy.
   ii) Extraction of hopeless posterior teeth.
   iii) Correction of local predisposing factors.
   iv) Urgent occlusal therapy.
   v) Treatment of gross caries and pulp symptoms.
c) Reassessment and definitive planning.
d) i) Root canal therapy.
   ii) Orthodontic therapy.
e) i) Stabilisation.
   ii) Temporisation.
f) Periodontal surgery.
g) Definitive conservation; fixed and removable prosthodontics.
h) Recall maintenance (*see* Chapter 16).

The advisability of elaborate forms of treatment (d–g) cannot be properly judged until after hygiene therapy. The need for reassessment after hygiene therapy, therefore, cannot be overstressed.

(a) Relief of Acute Symptoms

This may be a most rewarding way of gaining a patient's confidence and is usually essential before a patient can be expected to absorb further information or make decisions about less pressing matters.

(b) Hygiene Therapy and Simple Dental Treatment

(i) **Hygiene therapy.** This will include motivation and oral hygiene instruction, scaling, root planing and polishing (*see* Chapters 8 and 9).

(ii) **Extraction of hopeless posterior teeth.** Teeth which exhibit very advanced periodontal breakdown should be extracted. As a general rule, extractions, once decided upon, should be carried out early in treatment to facilitate healing of the periodontal tissues of adjacent teeth. This recommendation applies particularly to posterior teeth which rarely require immediate replacement with a denture. Extractions of anterior teeth, however, are often better postponed until surgical treatment has been completed, to avoid the adverse effect of a denture on the placement of periodontal dressing or the healing of an operated area.

(iii) **Correction of local predisposing factors.** At this stage, any obstacles to interdental cleaning, such as overhanging crown or filling margins, should be removed. This may necessitate replacement with a temporary restoration where the gingival condition is poor and the existing margin is subgingival. It may also be possible to modify the design of partial dentures in certain respects. This might include trimming the denture base away from gingival margins and relining with tissue conditioner to improve stability. Patients should have detailed denture hygiene instructions and should normally be advised to remove dentures at night. Consideration may also be given to recontouring teeth to decrease food impaction or facilitate cleaning. However, this may predispose to dentine sensitivity or caries.

(iv) **Urgent occlusal therapy.** Occlusal therapy in the form of splinting or occlusal adjustment is occasionally necessary during the early stages of treatment. Tooth mobility, however, is often less apparent following the completion of hygiene therapy. Only urgent occlusal therapy, therefore, should be carried out at this stage, since most forms of occlusal therapy have unwelcome side-effects. Occlusal adjustments, for example, are irreversible, destructive and, unless very precisely executed, are unlikely to have the desired long-term objective. Only teeth responsible for the most acute symptoms should ever be ground 'out of occlusion', as they will merely migrate or erupt again in an uncontrolled manner (*see* Chapters 4 and 15).

(v) **Treatment of gross caries and pulp symptoms.** This should be carried out for reasons of hygiene, to assess the feasibility of retaining and restoring such teeth and to avoid complications at a later stage.

(c) Reassessment and Definitive Planning

Following hygiene therapy, a time lapse of a few months is theoretically desirable before reassessment, to give some indication of the likelihood of long-term maintenance of oral hygiene by the patient. However, for practical purposes it is desirable to proceed with treatment planning as soon as maximal resolution of inflammation has taken place, about one month after the completion of hygiene therapy.

The definitive treatment plan will depend on the observed success of hygiene therapy, this being the most important prognostic indicator. Since prognosis is linked to the level of plaque control which can be sustained, planning is usually easier when motivation and cooperation are not in doubt. However, in practice, many patients, through lack of motivation or manual dexterity, fail to achieve satisfactory levels of plaque control, and it is consequently more difficult to arrive at a satisfactory treatment plan. The patient's aesthetic and functional expectations may need to be reduced and fulfilled by simpler forms of treatment. It may also be necessary to acknowledge that deterioration is likely and advise the patient accordingly. If resources are available, peridontal deterioration may be reduced by frequent meticulous professional tooth cleaning. The most advanced lesions, however, are less likely to respond even to scrupulously executed débridement.

Many patients will require some planning for edentulousness. Thus, it may be necessary to offset the deterioration which will result from wearing a transitional partial denture when oral hygiene is poor, against the advantages of a period of adaptation before a complete denture becomes inevitable.

One must be wary of being persuaded to carry out treatment which is contrary to one's professional judgement, and also of using limited clinical resources for treatment which has a poor prognosis.

Radiographs should be available and surveyed study casts will frequently be of benefit. The periodontal charting (Appendix I) should be completed with details of probing depths, mobility and furcation lesions, and comparison with earlier charting will give some indication of progress. Scrutiny of the chart, study casts and radiographs will allow decisions to be made about the feasibility of retaining teeth affected by advanced lesions, the need for surgery and the design of partial prostheses. Frequently, a number of options will be available and these must be discussed with the patient so that a step-by-step, detailed treatment plan may be formulated.

It is one of the ironies of periodontal treatment that those patients who show themselves to be willing and able to maintain a high standard of oral hygiene may be rewarded with more treatment and, in particular, periodontal surgery. Surgery is only justified for patients with good plaque control and any temptation to 'improve' a periodontium surgically and work on plaque control later must be resisted, particularly as research has shown that rapid loss of attachment can be expected if plaque accumulation occurs after surgery (Nyman *et al.*, 1977).

At this stage it must be decided which teeth are to be retained and an attempt should be made to maintain functional occlusal units if possible, i.e. teeth in opposition. It may be advisable to seek other specialist advice at this stage, particularly prosthodontic and orthodontic. If the teeth or periodontal conditions in the upper arch are poor, a complete upper denture opposed by natural lower teeth may constitute a satisfactory solution. On the other hand, a complete lower denture opposed by natural upper teeth is rarely acceptable and considerable effort should be made to avoid this eventuality. This is because the relatively poor support and retention of a complete lower denture, in opposition to a natural upper dentition, results in mucosal trauma and, simultaneously, risks accelerating resorption of the lower residual alveolar ridge.

It must also be decided whether it is necessary (or desirable) to replace missing teeth, and the possible designs of bridgework or partial denture should be considered at this stage. Orthodontic treatment should be considered, to restore the alignment of migrated teeth or to facilitate provision of a bridge or partial denture. Generally, orthodontic treatment should follow thorough scaling and establishment of good plaque control, but precede surgical treatment.

(d) Root Canal and Orthodontic Therapy

(i) **Root canal therapy.** If a combined lesion should affect the periodontal and pulpal tissues, it will be necessary to eliminate the pulpal disease in the first instance. Attempts at periodontal treatment are otherwise likely to fail because of the discharge from the infected or necrotic pulp. Moreover, where the lesion in the periodontal tissues is no more than a sinus, arising from the apex or from an accessory or lateral root canal, complete resolution of the combined lesion may be achieved by root canal therapy alone (Chapter 12).

Root canal therapy will be required for teeth with furcation lesions prior to root separation. This subject is considered in greater detail in Chapter 11.

(ii) **Orthodontic therapy.** Orthodontic treatment for teeth affected by periodontitis should be carried out only after thorough subgingival débridement. Failure to observe this important principle will subject the patient to the risk of an acute periodontal abscess when the pocket wall is compressed by the plaque-infected root surface.

Anterior teeth which have migrated as a result of periodontitis are frequently subjected to orthodontic treatment to achieve realignment. It must be appreciated, however, that subtle changes in anterior tooth position may occur which prevent straightforward retraction of the migrated tooth from achieving a perfect result. For example, as an upper incisor drifts forward and loses contact with its opponent, over-eruption of both teeth may occur to restore contact between them and form a barrier against palatal movement of the upper tooth. Elaborate orthodontic treatment, which might include intrusion of teeth in both arches, would then be necessary. On the other hand, it is sometimes possible to create space by grinding, although this does not give an ideal cosmetic result.

Fortunately, a number of migrated upper anterior teeth are associated with an anterior open bite owing to soft-tissue activity and realignment can be achieved without difficulty. Provided space can be created to accommodate a malaligned tooth, tooth movement is a simple matter which can be achieved in a short time because of the reduction in supporting tissues which has taken place.

Orthodontic therapy for the periodontal patient may also be indicated: to allow the achievement of a normal lip seal where protruding upper incisors are affected by 'mouth-breathing gingivitis'; to relieve deep traumatic overbite; to realign teeth partially excluded from the arch and suffering gingival recession as a result of this; to correct tooth malalignment caused by severe fibrous gingival hyperplasia; and to 'upright' tilted molar teeth.

A very important consideration, prior to orthodontic treatment for teeth with reduced periodontal support, is the means by which these teeth may be permanently retained in their new position, since it would seem prudent to anticipate a need for permanent retention. Indeed, the provision of permanent retention may be far more complex than the orthodontic treatment itself.

Anterior tooth migration, deep traumatic overbite and splinting after tooth movement are discussed in greater detail in Chapter 15.

(e) Stabilisation and Temporisation

(i) **Stabilisation.** Stabilisation may be regarded as a form of occlusal therapy and may be achieved by occlusal adjustment or splinting (*see* Chapter 15). Teeth which have been subjected to orthodontic movement will often require splinting. Likewise, it is occasionally necessary to splint teeth which are exceptionally mobile to avoid the risk of accidental avulsion during or immediately after surgery. Splinting may also be advisable where very mobile teeth cause discomfort.

(ii) **Temporisation.** Where it is anticipated that bridgework will ultimately replace a removable partial denture it is often helpful to carry out tooth preparation as far as possible and fit a temporary bridge prior to surgical intervention. By eliminating the partial denture, postoperative healing will be improved. It will frequently be necessary, however, to adjust the cervical margins and take the final impression of the crown preparations after surgery to take account of the longer clinical crowns. Where the fixed bridge is intended principally to stabilise mobile teeth, presurgical temporisation will have the added advantage of facilitating the surgical procedure as described in 'Stabilisation' (above).

(f) Periodontal Surgery

The need for surgery should be assessed on the basis of persistence of diseased sites, i.e. pockets which bleed on probing (*see* Chapter 5). Assuming optimal home care, surgery is justified if hygiene therapy fails to achieve resolution of inflammation and repair of the dentogingival junction. Thus, surgical treatment of shallow pockets (up to 3 mm) is not justified as direct access to such pockets for completion of scaling and root planing should present no problems and a shallow, physiological gingival sulcus should be obtainable. The surgical technique selected should not only allow access for scaling and root planing at the time of surgery but also result in a gingival contour which will allow plaque control afterwards and be acceptable cosmetically. Surgery may also be used to increase clinical crown length in order to facilitate restoration or improve artificial crown retention.

It is extremely important that the need for thorough home care in the long term is appreciated by the patient. Moreover, one must realise that patients cannot be relied on to achieve this without periodic supervision for reinforcement of motivation, oral hygiene instruction and scaling and polishing. Thus, an important part of treatment planning is the consideration of who will undertake responsibility for recall maintenance.

The information necessary for planning periodontal surgery is recorded on the chart in Appendix I. According to circumstances, surgery may be carried out in segments, quadrants or sides. The first surgical procedure should, if possible, be uncomplicated in order to preserve patient confidence. Before proceeding systematically with further surgery it is advisable to satisfy oneself that the anticipated result is likely to be achieved through optimal home care during healing. On the other hand, it may be difficult to maintain patient cooperation during an extended course of surgical treatment. There is, therefore, a good argument for attempting to complete the treatment schedule within the shortest convenient time. Such an approach should be reserved, however, for patients from whom good long-term plaque control can be confidently expected.

Oral hygiene techniques may need to be modified after each stage of surgery to take account of the inevitable change in gingival contour and area of exposed tooth surface. Dentine hypersensitivity may require treatment. Also, the exposure of more root surface may increase the risk of caries in a mouth with little recent experience of caries prior to surgery. Patients who appear to be developing root surface caries may benefit from periodic application of fluoride preparations, and should be counselled about dietary carbohydrate.

(g) Definitive Conservation; Fixed and Removable Prosthodontics

The highest-quality operative dentistry can be carried out only on teeth with good gingival conditions where gingival fluid flow and bleeding in response to minor trauma will be minimal. Gingival retraction, where necessary, can be carried out easily and this will result in better impressions, better-fitting crowns and less risk of subsequent gingival irritation or recession. Plastic restorations may be placed dry. The increase in crown length which results from reduction of marginal oedema and surgery will often make available additional undercut areas for partial-denture retention.

Replacement of missing teeth is not invariably necessary but may be required for aesthetic or functional reasons or as part of a transition to complete dentures. It may be desirable, also, to prevent further tipping, drifting or over-eruption, or to redistribute masticatory forces and achieve stabilisation of hypermobile teeth.

Where possible, a well-designed bridge is almost invariably preferable to a well-designed partial denture. Indeed, the latter may have an adverse effect on prognosis by enhancing plaque accumulation.

A partial denture can only be expected to improve the prognosis for remaining teeth if oral and denture hygiene are excellent, and if the denture makes a positive contribution towards more even distribution of occlusal forces, so limiting mobility or tendency to migrate. On the other hand, it may be advisable to provide partial dentures when further deterioration and tooth loss appear inevitable, in order that the patient may have some denture experience before provision of complete dentures. If possible, allowance should be made in the denture design for further tooth loss.

There are many patients in whom a premolar-to-premolar occlusion is acceptable both functionally and cosmetically (Kayser, 1981).

(h) Recall Maintenance

This is essential for a good prognosis to be achieved and must be seen as a long-term requirement. Prognosis is largely related to the level of plaque control which can be sustained by the patient at home. This will require periodic reinforcement. When failure does occur it is important to try to assess why, and not jump to the convenient conclusion that home care was inadequate.

REFERENCES

Kayser A. F. (1981). Shortened dental arches and oral function. *Journal of Oral Rehabilitation*; **8**: 457–62.

Nyman S., Lindhe J., Rosling B. (1977). Periodontal surgery in plaque-infected dentitions. *Journal of Clinical Periodontology*; **4**: 240–9.

FURTHER READING

Bradley R. E. (1972). Periodontal failures related to improper prognosis and treatment planning. *Dental Clinics of North America*; **16**: 33–46.

Lindhe J., Nyman S. (1975). The effect of plaque control and surgical pocket elimination on the establishment and maintenance of periodontal health. *Journal of Clinical Periodontology*; **2**: 67–78.

Ramfjord S. P., Ash M. M., Jr. (1979). Planning of periodontal therapy. In *Periodontology and Periodontics*. Ch. 12, pp. 313–34. Eastbourne: W. B. Saunders.

Wise M. D. (1985). Stability of gingival crest after surgery and before anterior crown placement. *Journal of Prosthetic Dentistry*; **53**: 20–3.

Chapter 8

Motivation and Instruction

The purpose of oral hygiene education is to establish behaviour which will prevent significant pathological effects of recurrent plaque accumulation and make the patient as independent as possible of professional support. This involves two related processes: motivation and instruction. Of these, the more exacting is motivation. It is relatively easy to teach the use of most hygiene aids but extremely difficult to ensure long-term compliance.

MOTIVATION

This aspect of patient education is often sadly neglected. When patients fail to reach adequate levels of plaque control, it is likely that what they require is not further instruction, but motivation. Most patients can remember relatively simple instructions given on previous visits, but many will lack the motivation to follow such instruction. Kegeles (1963) has suggested various steps which must be taken in an effort to motivate patients. These are referred to as the 'Kegeles Postulates' and they basically involve convincing the patient that a problem exists and that prevention is desirable. The postulates are listed as follows:

a) belief in susceptibility to the disease;
b) belief that the disease is undesirable;
c) belief that prevention is possible;
d) belief that prevention is desirable.

Sheiham (1979) has reviewed the scientific aspects of dental preventive behaviour while useful practical advice is given by Jacobson (1977). The reader is recommended to consult these articles to obtain an adequate appreciation of the problems of motivation. Some practical guidelines, however, are listed below.

a) Meet the patient at his own level, e.g. adult to adult. Avoid the risk of being condescending with some patients, or too deferential with others. Use terminology and language appropriate to the patient's education and background.

b)   Vary the approach to meet the patient's needs.

c)   Help the patient to recognise the benefits of prevention; for example, the avoidance of tooth loss; a reduction in operative dentistry; the avoidance of expensive restorative treatment; the preservation of appearance (manliness, femininity, etc.); the avoidance of toothache; self-approval; and the avoidance of bad breath.

d)   Do not create unfounded fears which may arouse feelings of resentment. Learning is more satisfactory in an atmosphere of trust and security.

e)   Do not build up unfounded hopes which cannot be fulfilled.

f)   Set patient objectives, which should consist of short-term goals such as: a reduction in disclosed plaque; a reduction in bleeding when brushing; a reduction in gingival swelling.

g)   Avoid offence, such as might be caused by telling the patient bluntly that his mouth is dirty.

h)   Stress every positive result at follow-up appointments and watch out for signs of discouragement.

i)   Explanatory leaflets may be useful, but should be supported by a personalised account of periodontal disease.

j)   Demonstration of periodontal disease in the patient's own mouth should have a satisfactory emotional impact. Plaque, gingivitis and pockets can easily be demonstrated. Disclosing agents may be useful initially but should not be relied upon for long-term maintenance of oral hygiene.

INSTRUCTION

There are a number of reasons for the limited effect of oral hygiene instruction in the past. For example, those giving it may not have been adequately trained and may often not have appreciated the problems involved even in one-to-one teaching. Moreover, many of the facts being taught have been inaccurate. For example, the idea that an apple or raw carrot may clean the teeth has been hallowed by time, and yet there is abundant evidence that fibrous foodstuffs do not remove plaque from any of the areas of the dentition most prone to caries or periodontal disease. Dental health education must be founded on scientific knowledge.

In recent years, the need for oral hygiene instruction to be given at the chairside has been questioned. Glavind *et al.* (1985) have shown that a self-instructional manual may be as effective as and less time consuming than chairside instruction by dental personnel.

Frequency of Tooth Cleaning

The prevention of chronic periodontal disease involves the thorough removal of plaque, sufficiently frequently to prevent pathological effects arising from recurrent plaque formation. It is known from a number of research reports, reviewed by Jenkins (1983), that many individuals will maintain gingival health by thorough plaque removal once every two days but that, to control gingivitis, rather than prevent its onset, more frequent plaque removal will be necessary.

To select a suitable cleaning frequency, one must take account not only of the existing periodontal condition, but also individual variations in plaque accumulation and predisposition to gingivitis and caries. Such considerations would indicate a brushing frequency for most individuals of twice daily, morning and night.

The thoroughness of plaque removal, however, is an important factor, since careless tooth cleaning will result in certain tooth surfaces consistently being missed. It is often prudent, therefore, to advise the patient that, however often he chooses to clean his teeth, he should do it thoroughly at least once a day when he can give tooth cleaning his undivided attention.

Toothbrushing

The brush. There is little scientific evidence to support particular toothbrush designs. Reason dictates, however, that a brush which is too large will not adequately fit into all areas of the dentition, whereas one which is too small will involve an unacceptably long time for brushing. Consequently, a brush head approximately one inch long for adult use seems reasonable with an appropriately smaller head for children. Multitufted, soft-filament nylon brushes are most widely accepted at the present time.

The paste. Toothpaste seems to make little contribution to the removal of plaque by brushes and other aids. The abrasive property of toothpaste, however, keeps the pellicle layer thin and prevents the accumulation of surface stains.

Technique. Many techniques for brushing teeth have been described and recommended with little evidence to support them. Various techniques are described by Greene (1966). Unfortunately, an incongruous situation has arisen where different authorities recommend different techniques and advise against others.

The Bass technique, or some modification of it, is probably regarded, worldwide, as the simplest and most efficient. The previously popular 'roll' technique has received unfavourable comment in a number of recent research reports, reviewed by Jenkins (1983). The Bass technique has the advantage of reaching into the gingival sulcus (Fig 8.1), while the 'roll' technique requires more manipulative skill and, especially in the presence of inflammatory swelling of the marginal gingiva, may miss the crevicular portion of the tooth (Fig. 8.2).

Although the Bass technique is suitable for teaching to individuals whose oral hygiene is poor, many patients require

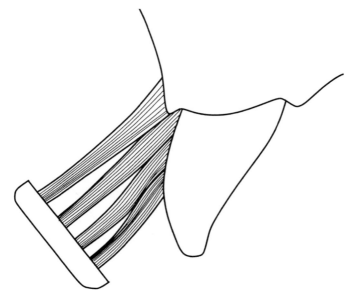

Fig. 8.1 *The Bass method of toothbrushing. The bristles are directed into the gingival sulcus at 45° angle to the long axis of the teeth and the brush is activated with a short back-and-forth vibrating motion.*

little brushing instruction, having evolved a technique of their own.

Although some toothbrushing techniques are designed specifically to remove plaque from interdental areas, it is doubtful whether any method of brushing will remove proximal surface plaque to a significant extent. For this reason, the use of other interdental cleaning devices is highly recommended.

Advice on brushing should follow an examination of the mouth and should relate to specific problems. Such evidence as exists would suggest that it is not only the actual brushing stroke which the patient uses which matters but also a thorough and methodical approach. Many patients have a poor knowledge of the anatomy of their own dentitions and do not fully appreciate how retentive plaque is or the degree of brushing required to remove it. Few patients, consequently, realise the time needed to brush the dentition adequately. Few people spend more than 30 seconds on toothbrushing and this is totally inadequate for the individual with average manipulative skill. Advice to extend the brushing period might, in fact, be more beneficial to many patients than dwelling unduly on a particular technique.

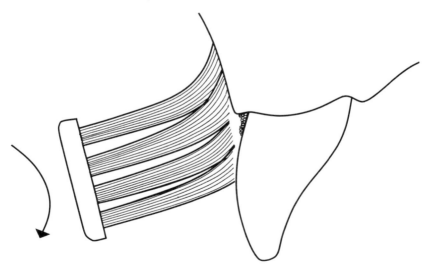

Fig. 8.2   *The 'roll technique' of toothbrushing. The bristles are applied to the attached gingiva pointing apically, then swept in a coronal direction, crossing the tooth at right angles. Plaque in the crevice region will be 'protected' from the bristles by a thickened marginal gingiva.*

Special brushes. In certain cases, where patient motivation seems adequate, the use of special brushes such as the single-tufted brush ('interspace brush') may be recommended. This device may be put to use in a multitude of ways: to clean malaligned teeth and teeth affected by localised gingival recession; to clean the proximal surfaces of teeth adjacent to a saddle area; to clean the distal surface of the last molar tooth; and, as an adjunct to interdental woodsticks, to compensate for the failure of the latter to remove plaque from lingual embrasures.

Whereas there appears to be little value in recommending the electric toothbrush to the average patient, such brushes can be of value to physically or, possibly, mentally handicapped patients.

Interdental Cleaning

Patients can rarely achieve periodontal health without an interdental cleaning aid such as floss or woodsticks. Efficiently used, floss is undoubtedly more effective in the removal of proximal surface plaque than is the woodstick. Additionally, floss is capable of removing plaque from subgingival surfaces and from lingual embrasures, whereas woodsticks are not. The use of floss, however, is time consuming and calls for a degree of motivation and dexterity not found in all individuals. In general, the use of woodsticks takes less time than floss, calls for less manual dexterity and, consequently, may require slightly less motivation. It may, in some cases, be preferable to accept regular use of woodsticks than infrequent use of floss. On the other hand, the woodstick is effective only when sufficient interdental space is available to accommodate it.

It should be remembered that various modifications of dental floss exist, such as dental tape and Super Floss®, each of which may be of advantage in some cases. Whether waxed or unwaxed floss is used seems largely a matter of personal choice, although patients with heavy interproximal restorations may prefer waxed floss, since it is less prone to shredding.

Interdental brushes ('bottle brushes') are important devices since they are essential to the long-term success of surgical procedures which result in a large area of interdental gingival recession. In this situation, there is often a proximal furrow in the root which cannot be adequately cleaned by floss or sticks but which will accommodate an interdental brush well (Fig. 8.3).

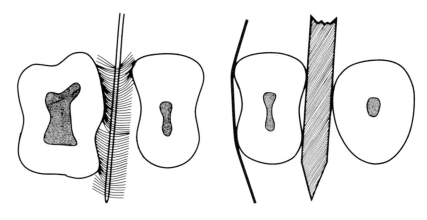

Fig. 8.3   *Interdental aids: failure of woodpoints and dental floss to clean proximal root furrows, compared with the interdental brush, which enters these root surface concavities when correctly angulated.*

Some debate has existed regarding the age at which interdental cleaning should be established. Young children are unlikely to possess either the manual dexterity or the motivation to practise interdental cleaning. However, interdental cleaning should certainly be recommended once the permanent dentition is established (other than the third molar teeth) in the early teenage years. At this age, interdental gingival recession is unlikely to have occurred and dental floss will be the only suitable interdental aid.

Mouthwashes

The most effective chemical antiplaque agent available at the present time is chlorhexidine gluconate. Chlorhexidine is a cationic bisbiguanide antiseptic which possesses the property of adsorption to oral surfaces, notably enamel, and of gradual release to exert a prolonged bactericidal effect. It has a fairly broad antibacterial spectrum.

Used twice daily in 0·2% solution, it is unmatched by any other commercially available mouthwash and will effectively prevent plaque accumulation and gingivitis. However, when used as a mouthwash, it will not penetrate subgingivally and is unlikely to have any worthwhile effect where gingival or periodontal pockets are present. Furthermore, it has an unpleasant taste, interferes with taste appreciation and discolours teeth and restorations. Stain removal from proximal surfaces can be extremely time consuming. These factors limit the periodontal use of chlorhexidine mouthwash to a few specific situations:

a) postoperative plaque control;
b) plaque control in handicapped patients;
c) patients with desquamative gingivitis;
d) patients with intermaxillary fixation;
e) patients with primary herpetic stomatitis;
f) after acute necrotising ulcerative gingivitis, when sensitivity and poor gingival contours inhibit mechanical tooth cleaning.

Chlorhexidine mouthwash used during the initial phase of hygiene therapy will mask the effects of personal mechanical plaque control and will make proper evaluation of the patient's efforts impossible. Use of chlorhexidine during hygiene therapy is, therefore, advised only on the rare occasion when gingivitis is so severe that effective mechanical oral hygiene is impossible and then the drug must be withdrawn at the earliest opportunity.

Recent work has shown that a 400 ml solution of 0·02% (one-tenth mouthwash concentration), delivered to the teeth from a pulsating oral irrigator once daily, may be the most effective method of achieving supragingival plaque control. This regime enables the chemical to be well distributed to all tooth surfaces and allows a lower concentration to be used, which helps to minimise the local side-effects.

CONCLUDING REMARKS

Oral hygiene instruction will rarely produce the desired result after only one lesson, and usually many visits are necessary. Once toothbrushing is mastered, other appropriate aids should be introduced gradually and the patient should be asked at each visit to demonstrate his toothcleaning skills at the chairside, while the clinician observes his progress and offers help where necessary. Visits for oral hygiene instruction should continue until the patient has reached his peak level of performance. This, unfortunately, may not be sufficient to ensure gingival health in many cases.

Personal mechanical plaque control, and indeed chemical

antiplaque agents, can prevent gingivitis and probably resolve inflammation in its early stages. Their effectiveness in preventing the extension of pre-existing periodontal disease is, however, questionable. Professional subgingival cleaning is, therefore, an essential part of treatment where pockets are present.

REFERENCES

Glavind L., Christensen H., Pedersen E., Rosendahl H., Attstrom R. (1985). Oral hygiene instruction in general dental practice by means of self-teaching manuals. *Journal of Clinical Periodontology*; **12**: 27–34.

Greene J. C. (1966). Oral health care for prevention and control of periodontal disease. In *World Workshop in Periodontics* (Ramfjord S. P., Kerr D. A., Ash M. M., eds.) p. 339. Ann Arbor: University of Michigan Press.

Jacobson L. (1977). Does your message satisfy your patients' needs? *Dental Health*; **16**: 11–16.

Jenkins W. M. M. (1983). The prevention and control of chronic periodontal disease. In *Prevention of Dental Disease* (Murray J. J., ed.) Ch. 9. Oxford: Oxford University Press.

Kegeles S. S. (1963). Why people seek dental care: the test of conceptual formulation. *Journal of Health and Human Behaviour*; **4**: 166–73.

Sheiham A. (1979). The prevention and control of periodontal disease. *Dental Health*; **18**: 7–20.

FURTHER READING

Addy M. (1986). Chlorhexidine compared with other locally delivered antimicrobials. A short review. *Journal of Clinical Periodontology*; **13**: 957–64.

Blinkhorn A. S., Fox B., Holloway P. J. (1983). *Notes on Dental Health Education*. Edinburgh: Scottish Health Education Group, and London: Health Education Authority.

Ramfjord S. P., Ash J. J. (1979). Oral hygiene. In *Periodontology and Periodontics*. Ch. 16. Eastbourne: W. B. Saunders.

Chapter 9

Scaling and Root Planing

Effective scaling and root planing is fundamental to the success of all aspects of periodontal treatment. Expertise in this field is essential for all those involved in the management of periodontal disease. Much of this chapter applies equally to the scaling and root planing procedures which accompany most forms of surgical therapy, although the comments which follow are primarily about non-surgical débridement.

OBJECTIVES

The objectives of tooth surface instrumentation can be clearly stated thus: (1) to remove supragingival accretions leaving a smooth and polished surface which will facilitate rapid and simple day-to-day plaque removal by the patient; (2) to remove subgingival root surface irritants, i.e. plaque, calculus and pathologically altered cementum, to allow healing in the soft-tissue pocket wall and, if possible, to achieve new epithelial attachment with the formation of a physiological gingival sulcus.

Scaling and root planing are fully effective only at surfaces which are readily accessible to instrumentation. Recent research, however, has shown that there is no certain magnitude of initial probing depth above which non-surgical instrumentation is ineffective, provided sufficient skill and perseverance are applied. Even when subgingival instrumentation is incomplete, perhaps owing to insufficient access, and healing of the pocket wall is not achieved, the progress of periodontal disease may still be retarded until a periodontopathic flora becomes re-established. This may take several months (Listgarten *et al.*, 1978).

TERMINOLOGY

Scaling

The term 'scaling' refers to the physical removal from the tooth surface of accretions, notably plaque, calculus and stained pellicle.

Root Planing

Root planing involves the removal of pathologically altered cementum and smoothing of the root surface. It will also achieve removal of plaque and calculus which have become embedded in surface irregularities. The degree of root smoothness which is achieved may not be of biological importance but it gives the best clinical indication that calculus and altered cementum have been removed. The exposure of root dentine, although not intended, may, nevertheless, be unavoidable.

Scaling and root planing are best considered as a single treatment procedure since scaling inevitably removes some cementum, and root planing will remove plaque and calculus deposits which are embedded within surface irregularities.

Curettage

Subgingival scaling and root planing is sometimes referred to as 'root curettage', although this may lead to confusion with the expression 'subgingival curettage', which is reserved for scraping and removal of soft tissue from within the pocket. A certain amount of subgingival curettage is unavoidable during scaling and root planing, particularly when curettes are used. Nevertheless, it has been shown that purposeful subgingival curettage is not a worthwhile procedure, since the results achieved by scaling and root planing with subgingival curettage are no better than those obtained by scaling and root planing alone (Hill *et al.*, 1981). The subject of subgingival curettage will not, therefore, be discussed further.

DETECTION OF CALCULUS

Supragingival calculus is easily identified when present in large deposits, and trace amounts can be readily visualised by drying the teeth with an air syringe. This is a useful way of assessing the adequacy of supragingival scaling.

Subgingival calculus may be visualised to some extent by distending the pocket orifice with a flat plastic instrument or by gently blowing air into the pocket. Subgingival calculus may also be demonstrated using a fine probe and, indeed, the tactile sense has to be relied upon for detection of deep calculus.

Radiographs are unreliable for calculus detection since only large radio-opaque deposits will be visible, and then only on proximal surfaces when the beam angulation is suitable.

TREATMENT PROCEDURES

The approach to scaling will clearly vary, depending on the extent of deposits and distribution and depth of pockets. Generally, it is advisable to complete the supragingival scaling in the first appointment to facilitate the patient's personal plaque control. At the following visit, approximately one week later, substantial resolution of superficial inflammation should be apparent. Subgingival instrumentation, ideally, should not be initiated until the patient is capable of performing adequate plaque control. This means that anterior teeth will probably be ready for instrumentation before posterior teeth where adequate plaque control takes longer to learn. Subgingival débridement is likely to be much more time consuming than supragingival scaling, in view of the greater hardness and tenacity of subgingival calculus and the need for subsequent root planing. The operator should adopt a segmental approach, each tooth in the chosen segment being scaled and root planed to *completion* before moving to the next segment. This approach is preferable to the 'circuit' method where the entire mouth is part scaled at each appointment, increments of calculus being removed at each circuit until (hopefully!) none remains. The preferred, segmental method ensures maximal thoroughness and efficiency and it facilitates the use of local anaesthesia where necessary. This latter approach, however, is not suitable for pockets which are sites of an intense inflammatory process since there is a great risk that the zone of inflamed connective tissue, apical to the epithelial attachment, will be penetrated by the scaling instrument. If the scaling procedure extends beyond the base of the pocket in this way, permanent loss of connective tissue attachment may occur. Accordingly, where the base of the pocket cannot confidently be identified by the operator and where bleeding on probing is profuse, instrumentation should be a two-stage process; the initial subgingival scaling being carried out at a relatively superficial level. The next scaling session should be postponed for about one month to allow for the establishment of new gingival collagen which will provide a landmark for the extension of further scaling and root planing.

Scaling will be greatly facilitated by the chairside assistant providing a 'washed field' with aspiration. Local anaesthetics are often necessary, since pain may otherwise be experienced from sensitive root surfaces and the investing soft tissue. Local anaesthesia should not be used, however, when severe periodontal inflammation is present since there will already be a risk of over-extending the field of scaling as described above, and elimination of pain responses by local anaesthetic will increase this risk.

When scaling and root planing is completed, all accessible surfaces should be polished with a fine abrasive polishing paste to reduce surface roughness as far as possible, so minimising subsequent plaque accumulation. Polishing pastes which are sufficiently abrasive to remove stains will also remove tooth substance and leave a rough surface. Coarse pastes should, therefore, be used only on surfaces where stain removal is necessary, and this should be followed by a polish with a fine-particle paste.

Buccal and lingual surfaces are best polished with a rubber cup, while proximal surfaces may be polished to some extent by hand with woodpoints or dental tape.

INSTRUMENTS AND MATERIALS

Hand Instruments

'Scalers' is a generic term for the instruments used in scaling and root planing. These are produced by a large number of manufacturers, and instruments of the same type may vary greatly in size, shape and construction.

The head of a scaling instrument has a shank and a working tip of stainless steel, carbon steel or tungsten carbide.

Stainless steel heads become blunt quickly and should be sharpened after every use. They are, however, easily sharpened by a person familiar with the procedure. Carbon steel, too, is easily sharpened and retains its edge longer than stainless steel but discolouration and corrosion tend to occur during sterilisation. Tungsten carbide tips, being harder than steel, maintain their edge much longer. When a tungsten carbide tip does become dull, it will not be readily amenable to sharpening.

Scalers are classified as chisels, sickles, hoes and curettes (Fig. 9.1).

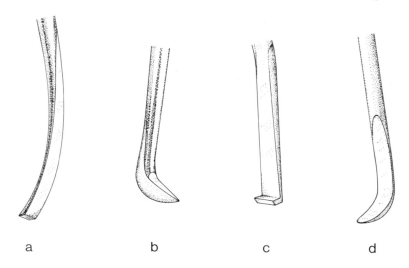

a   b   c   d

Fig. 9.1 *Scalers:* (a) *chisel,* (b) *'straight' sickle,* (c) *hoe and* (d) *curette.*

Push scaler (chisel scaler). This is used for removing calculus from interproximal surfaces of mandibular anterior teeth. It is used from the labial aspect with a pen grasp and controlled push, with the fulcrum finger placed on the labial surfaces of adjacent teeth. This is a very effective instrument but it must be seated with extreme care to avoid gouging the root surface with one of the sharp corners.

Sickle scalers. These have two cutting edges on a curved blade converging to a sharp point. They are used for supragingival scaling of proximal tooth surfaces. The cutting edge should be pulled coronally and, because there is an edge on both sides of the blade, they can be used on the distal aspect of one tooth and the mesial aspect of the adjacent tooth by the same basic approach with a slightly altered blade angle. Because of its design and size, the sickle scaler is not adaptable for subgingival use. Sickle scalers are available with curved shanks for use on posterior teeth.

The Hygienist range of scalers include a group of sickle scalers with heads which are finer and more flexible, and are particularly suited to teeth in close contact.

Jaquette scalers have a straight blade, but are classified as a type of sickle.

Periodontal hoes. These have a cutting edge, set at right angles to the shank. A set of four different hoes are required to give access to all surfaces. Hoes are used to remove supra- and subgingival calculus, although they are not very manoeuvrable within periodontal pockets. They are much more useful when surgical access has been obtained. They are used with a coronally directed stroke and, like chisels, must be properly seated to avoid gouging the root surface with the corner of the blade. MacFarlane pattern hoes have finer blades which make them more suited to subgingival scaling. They also have a slightly curved blade which reduces the likelihood of soft-tissue trauma.

Curettes. These instruments have two cutting edges and a curved continuous spoon-shaped working end. The back of the instrument is rounded. These instruments are unique amongst scalers in having no sharp corners or points which can gouge the root surface or lacerate the gingiva. The curette is, therefore, the instrument of choice for removing deep subgingival calculus and root planing.

Curettes are supplied in pairs. A very large number of designs are available which vary according to length and shape of the shank, blade design and size. The variations permit the use of the instrument in all mouth areas; for example, the more acute the angle of the shank, the more suited will be the instrument for posterior teeth.

Ultrasonic Scalers

Many units are available with a wide range of specifications. They fall generally into one of two categories.

Magnetostrictive (electromagnetic) units. This is the traditional type of unit. It comprises a working tip, coupled to a stack of ferromagnetic metal in a high-frequency magnetic field. The 'stack' undergoes alternate expansion and contraction in response to application and removal of the magnetic field at a rate of about 25 000 cycles per second, and this results in a similar vibration frequency of the working tip. The amplitude of the vibratory movement is about 0·006–0·1 mm. The working tip describes a linear, rectilinear or elliptical movement.

Much of the energy produced by the ultrasonic machine is dissipated in the form of heat. This is reduced by water, passing through the tip, being directed to the working areas. Besides serving a cooling function, the water is atomised into tiny vacuum bubbles, which collapse with the release of energy and help to clear the field of loose debris. The formation of vacuum bubbles has been described as 'cavitation' and was once believed to be an important factor in dislodging calculus from the teeth. It is now known, however, that deposits must be touched with the instrument and are thus removed mechanically.

Piezoelectric units. This is a new generation of ultrasonic unit in which the magnetostriction stack is replaced by a quartz crystal mechanism. When an oscillating voltage is applied, the crystal swings to either side of its rest position, resulting in high-frequency tip vibration. Less heat is produced and, therefore, less coolant is necessary, so reducing the need for aspiration. These devices are very efficient although easily damaged if dropped.

Air-driven Scalers

Air-driven units work by compressed air activating a vibrating rod. These units are not truly ultrasonic but work at sonic frequencies. They have the advantage of fitting readily into any dental unit with a compressed-air supply and, therefore, are relatively inexpensive. According to recent research, there may be little difference in clinical efficacy between air-driven (sonic) scalers and ultrasonic scalers although patient acceptance of air-driven scalers may be poorer.

ULTRASONIC INSTRUMENTATION

The power control adjusts the actual power generated by the oscillator and the amplitude of tip movements. The lowest possible setting, consistent with satisfactory resonance, should be used to reduce trauma. Tuning may be automatic, but if a tuning control is provided, this should be used to adjust the frequency of the oscillator until a 'hiss' is heard and the water spray atomises well. Because of the aerosol, a face mask should be worn and eye protection is also advisable.

The patient's medical history should be reviewed since ultrasonic scaling is contraindicated for patients who:

a)   are carriers of the hepatitis B virus, since the widened

droplet zone, caused by the aerosol of the instrument, may increase the likelihood of spread of the virus;
b) have a cardiac pacemaker, since it is suggested that the ultrasonic vibrations might upset the pacemaker rhythm.

Technique

A pen grasp should be used with the handpiece and the working tip applied as nearly parallel to the long axis of the tooth as possible and, at worst, at no more than 15° to the tooth surface. With an angulation greater than 15°, the root surface may be scratched.

The tip should be kept in motion at all times to avoid overheating any part of the tooth surface. It is essential to ensure that the water spray reaches the operating area. A light brushing type of stroke should be used with the minimum of pressure.

Indications

It has long been accepted that the ultrasonic unit can accomplish supragingival scaling at least as quickly as with hand instruments. Furthermore, the cleansing effect of the water jet is a particular advantage when scaling a dirty mouth or one in which gingival bleeding is profuse. Patients usually experience less pain during ultrasonic instrumentation. This is a particularly important consideration in the treatment of acute necrotising ulcerative gingivitis.

The use of the ultrasonic unit subgingivally has not met with as much general acceptance, since the operator is unable to see the field, tactile sensation is poor and root surfaces cannot be planed. Nevertheless, numerous reports (e.g. Badersten *et al.*, 1984) indicate that the ultrasonic instrument, compared with hand instrumentation, is equally effective in removing subgingival plaque and calculus and the periodontal response to instrumentation is similar with both methods. That, together with the fact that most patients and operators prefer the ultrasonic technique, would suggest that these devices have a much greater application than was once thought to be the case.

Although an ultrasonic device will remove contaminated cementum, it does not leave the root surface smooth. In practice, this drawback appears to be unimportant subgingivally, although a rough supragingival tooth surface is likely to accumulate more plaque than a smooth one, which is more amenable to home cleaning.

POCKET IRRIGATION

It is common practice after subgingival instrumentation to irrigate pockets with a 0·2% solution of chlorhexidine. While there may be some slight benefit from the mechanical flushing effect, there is *no* clinical evidence of a significant chemical effect on the subgingival flora (*see* Chapter 20).

HEALING AFTER SCALING AND ROOT PLANING

Following subgingival instrumentation, bacterial remnants will tend to be washed out of the pocket by blood and gingival fluid. Within a few hours of scaling and root planing, an acute inflammatory reaction occurs in the soft-tissue pocket wall. Remnants of pocket epithelium will proliferate and the pocket wall will be fully epithelialised within two days. Involution of pocket epithelium will occur giving rise to new junctional epithelium. After five days, epithelial reattachment will commence at the apical extremity of the pocket, and progress coronally until, under conditions of ideal plaque control, epithelial reattachment will be complete in 14 days and a new gingival sulcus will be formed near to the crest of the gingiva. Some shrinkage of gingiva will occur owing to loss of oedema. The formation of functionally orientated collagen, to replace granulation tissue, tends to lag behind the healing of the dentoepithelial junction, immature collagen not appearing until after three weeks.

The above healing sequence will occur only following adequate subgingival débridement which, according to Waerhaug (1978), cannot confidently be expected except in pockets less than 3 mm in depth. Complete repair of the dentoepithelial junction is also dependent on effective supragingival plaque control during and after the healing phase.

Incomplete subgingival débridement will allow persistence of inflammation and, in due course, recolonisation of the subgingival root surface from bacterial residues. Likewise, failure to prevent supragingival plaque accumulation will lead to down-growth of bacterial plaque, which will halt the process of coronally advancing epithelial reattachment.

Traditionally, pockets which do not respond adequately to a reasonable amount of subgingival débridement are subjected to surgery if home care is good. Surgery will lead to a reduction in pocket depth and will arrest the lost of connective tissue attachment so long as adequate maintenance care is provided. In recent years, however, it has been shown that scaling and root planing meticulously performed for advanced periodontitis will achieve results comparable to surgical therapy, again assuming that adequate maintenance care is provided. (Pihlstrom *et al.*, 1983; Badersten *et al.*, 1984; Lindhe *et al.*, 1984; Ramfjord *et al.*, 1987). Non-surgical scaling and root planing, however, as a definitive procedure in deep pockets, is very time consuming as the aforementioned studies reveal.

Badersten *et al.* (1984) devoted, on average, approximately 11 minutes per single-rooted tooth to scaling and root planing with hand instruments. This could be reduced to approximately 10 minutes per single-rooted tooth when ultrasonic instruments were employed. The teeth in this study had pocket depths of 4–12 mm.

The regime of Ramfjord *et al.* (1987) included 5–8 hours (4–6 appointments) of the dental hygienist's time in scaling, root planing and oral hygiene instruction, then further scaling and root planing by a periodontist, followed by recall prophylaxis at three-month intervals. These patients had moderate to severe periodontitis.

Pihlstrom *et al.* (1983) took 6–8 hours (3–4 appointments) to administer scaling, root planing and oral hygiene instruction for patients with moderate to advanced periodontitis, followed by recall prophylaxis every 3–4 months during the experimental period. Each recall lasted 1 hour.

Lindhe *et al.* (1984) took 3–4 appointments per quadrant to complete scaling and root planing and followed this with three-monthly recall prophylaxis for a group of patients with advanced periodontal disease.

From the foregoing account, it should be apparent that scaling and root planing of deep pockets is neither a quick and easy nor an inexpensive alternative to periodontal surgery.

The aforementioned studies also reveal that, although healthy periodontal conditions were achieved by scaling and root planing, with or without surgical access, shallow pockets (less than 4 mm probing depth) after treatment showed some minor attachment loss. Deep pockets (more than 6 mm probing depth), on the other hand, showed some gain in *clinical* attachment after treatment. In all probability, some connective tissue fibre attachment would be destroyed inadvertently by instrumentation in both categories of pocket. However, the connective tissue attachment loss after treatment of deep pockets would be masked by the resistance to probing produced by a long epithelial attachment and its supporting gingival connective tissue, as well as by bone-fill in certain cases. Pockets of intermediate depth (4–6 mm) maintain their clinical attachment levels following successful surgical or non-surgical treatment.

CONCLUDING REMARKS

From the many longitudinal studies published in recent years it now appears that the 'critical probing depth' at which non-surgical instrumentation provides more favourable healing than flap procedures may be greater than previously considered (Lindhe *et al.*, 1982). Surgery, however, is often required for the definitive treatment of deep tortuous pockets and the management of furcation lesions. Furthermore, in the non-surgical treatment of infrabony pockets, bone-fill may not occur to the same extent as may be expected from surgical débridement and the formation of a coagulum within the bone defect.

REFERENCES

Badersten A., Nilveus R., Egelberg J. (1984). Effects of non-surgical periodontal therapy. II Severely advanced periodontitis. *Journal of Clinical Periodontology*; 11: 63–76.

Hill R. W., Ramfjord S. P., Morrison E. C., *et al.* (1981). Four types of periodontal treatment compared over two years. *Journal of Periodontology*; 52: 655–62.

Lindhe J., Socransky S. S., Nyman S., Haffajee A., Westfeldt E. (1982). 'Critical probing depths' in periodontal therapy. *Journal of Clinical Periodontology*; 9: 323–36.

Lindhe J., Westfelt E., Nyman S., Socransky S. S., Haffajee A. D. (1984). Long-term effect of surgical/non-surgical treatment of periodontal disease. *Journal of Clinical Periodontology*; 11: 448–58.

Listgarten M. A., Lindhe J., Helldén L. (1978). Effect of tetracycline and/or scaling on human periodontal disease. Clinical, micro-biological and histological observations. *Journal of Clinical Periodontology*; **5**: 246–71.

Pihlstrom B. L., McHugh R. B., Oliphant T. H., Ortiz-Campos C. (1983). Comparison of surgical and non-surgical treatment of periodontal disease. *Journal of Clinical Periodontology*; **10**: 524–41.

Ramfjord S. P., Caffesse R. G., Morrison E. C., *et al.* (1987). 4 modalities of periodontal treatment compared over 5 years. *Journal of Clinical Periodontology*; **14**: 445–52.

Waerhaug J. (1978). Healing of the dento-epithelial junction following sub-gingival plaque control. II. As observed on extracted teeth. *Journal of Periodontology*; **49**: 119–34.

FURTHER READING

Cercek J. F., Kiger R. D., Garrett S., Egelberg J. (1983). Relative effects of plaque control and instrumentation on the clinical parameters of human periodontal disease. *Journal of Clinical Periodontology*; **10**: 46–56.

Clark S. M., (1969). The ultrasonic dental unit—a guide for the clinical application of ultrasonics in dentistry and dental hygiene. *Journal of Periodontology*; **40**: 621–9.

Suppipat N. (1974). Ultrasonics in periodontics. *Journal of Clinical Periodontology*; **1**: 206–13.

Tabita P. V., Bissada N. F., Maybury J. E. (1981). Effectiveness of supra-gingival plaque control on the development of sub-gingival plaque and gingival inflammation in patients with moderate pocket depth. *Journal of Periodontology*; **52**: 88–93.

Waerhaug J. (1978). Healing of the dento–epithelial junction following sub-gingival plaque control. I. As observed in human biopsy material. *Journal of Periodontology*; **49**: 1–8.

Chapter 10

Periodontal Surgery

'Periodontal surgery' is a term which is usually reserved for procedures requiring the use of a scalpel. Surgical procedures in current use include:

a) gingivectomy—simply the removal of unwanted gingival tissue;
b) a flap procedure to improve access to the root surface for completion of root instrumentation in cases of advanced periodontitis;
c) mucogingival surgery to increase the width of attached gingiva.

For convenience, mucogingival surgery is described in Chapter 13. Only the gingivectomy procedure and flap surgery for periodontitis are discussed here. The reader's attention is drawn to the descriptions of structural changes during healing and the rationale of surgical treatment considered in Chapter 6.

THE GINGIVECTOMY PROCEDURE

Indications

Gingival hyperplasia. Mild gingival hyperplasia is common in simple gingivitis, particularly around crowded teeth or within relief areas of partial dentures. In its most severe form it is associated with systemic modifying factors (Chapter 3). Surgical removal of the enlarged tissues may be desirable: for cosmetic reasons; because of interference with occlusion; to facilitate operative dental surgery or prosthodontic work; in combination with a flap procedure for underlying periodontitis; or because the bulky gingiva appears to prevent adequate oral hygiene.

Hygiene therapy must be performed before considering gingival surgery. There are two principal reasons for this. Firstly, if good oral hygiene can be established, sufficient tissue shrinkage may occur to obviate the need for surgery. Secondly, dental plaque is an important aetiological factor in all forms of gingival hyperplasia and, unless good plaque control is achieved postoperatively, recurrent gingival enlargement is inevitable. By testing the patient's level of commitment and manual dexterity during a presurgical phase of hygiene therapy, the clinician will be able to predict the likely long-term outcome of treatment. In patients with persistently poor plaque control in spite of oral hygiene instruction, the clinician may decide that the problem is not sufficiently severe to justify the short-term advantage of gingivectomy. Very occasionally gingival hyperplasia is so severe that it is unreasonable to expect the patient to achieve good supragingival plaque control and surgery may proceed without the patient reaching the oral hygiene standards normally expected prior to surgical intervention.

It should be noted that surgical intervention is not justifiable for minor aberrations of gingival anatomy which are frequently present following resolution of gingival inflammation, but which do not usually prevent access to the cervical tooth region by appropriate oral hygiene aids.

Interdental soft-tissue craters. Gingivitis (particularly acute necrotising ulcerative gingivitis) and occasionally periodontitis may lead to the formation of crater-like depressions of the interdental gingiva. Furthermore, a similar deformity may develop following surgery for periodontitis if buccal and lingual flap margins fail to unite. In these various circumstances, access for cleaning proximal tooth surfaces may be poor and gingivectomy may be required to remove one or both soft-tissue crater margins.

Subgingival restoration margins. Restorations located below the gingival margin tend to promote subgingival plaque accumulation. Gingivectomy may be used to deliberately create gingival recession at these locations. This may result in a permanently located supragingival margin or may simply provide temporary access to insert a new restoration with a better marginal finish (Chapter 17).

Technique

Although there is a fine distinction to be drawn between the terms 'gingivoplasty' (surgical recontouring) and 'gingivectomy' (excision of gingival tissue), the latter will be adhered to for simplicity of discussion. Notwithstanding differences in terminology, the surgical procedures are the same and are illustrated in Figure 10.1. Following anaesthesia, a bevelled incision through the

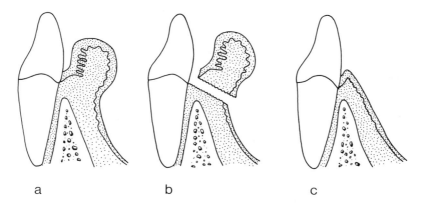

a   b   c

Fig. 10.1 *Gingivectomy.* (a) *Gingival hyperplasia;* (b) *bevelled incision;* (c) *formation of new marginal gingiva.*

gingiva is directed at the base of the pocket. The detached gingiva is removed and the exposed tooth surface instrumented. A periodontal dressing is adapted to the wound surface and left in place for one week to give protection and minimise discomfort. In addition, by occupying the interdental space, it prevents the formation of excessive granulation tissue, and so encourages good postoperative contour.

In the surgical treatment of gross gingival hyperplasia, an open-wound gingivectomy may be combined with an under-mining flap operation to avoid the creation of a large connective tissue wound.

Healing after Gingivectomy

From the second postoperative day onwards, epithelial cells migrate over the wound surface from the wound margin towards the tooth at the rate of about 0·5 mm per day. Epithelialisation, therefore, is barely complete by the time of dressing removal, and keratinisation takes a further two weeks. Proliferation of fibroblasts adjacent to the wound surface occurs, leading to coronal regrowth of tissue and the formation of a new free gingival unit by about the seventh postoperative day. The formation and maturation of collagen takes place from about the third week as a new epithelial attachment is formed. Complete healing of the gingivectomy wound takes about six weeks but minor dimensional changes may continue for several months.

The Gingivectomy Procedure in Treatment of Periodontitis

It will be apparent that, so far, no mention has been made of a possible role for gingivectomy in the treatment of periodontitis. In fact, there are a number of reasons why gingivectomy is not an appropriate approach to this problem.

Deep pockets of, say, 5 mm or more tend to be infrabony in nature and tend to extend beyond the mucogingival line. Clearly, a bevelled gingivectomy would not be helpful. It would not eliminate the pocket. It would cause an excessive amount of gingival recession and would not leave a functional width of attached gingiva. This, of course, has never been disputed.

Pockets of up to 3–4 mm which bleed or exude pus on probing should be considered accessible for non-surgical scaling or root planing.

Pockets of up to 3–4 mm which do not bleed or exude pus on probing do not require further treatment. Such non-inflamed pockets frequently result from successful instrumentation of the diseased root surface against which the overlying gingival tissues form a long epithelial attachment. Although inflammation disappears as healing progresses, in the past it was erroneously believed that 3–4 mm probing depths would mitigate against continued periodontal health. This was one of the principal reasons for advocating a gingivectomy procedure. Nowadays, gingivectomy in the treatment of periodontitis can be justified only where gingival hyperplasia and periodontitis coexist or where the gingiva has to be surgically recontoured during a flap operation to achieve a good postoperative gingival contour.

SURGICAL TREATMENT OF PERIODONTITIS

Objectives and Indications

The main objective of surgical intervention in the treatment of periodontitis is the provision of good access for the completion of scaling and root planing, thereby to create a physiological gingival sulcus and preserve connective tissue attachment.

Unlike hyperplastic gingivitis and acute necrotising ulcerative gingivitis, periodontitis is a disease usually with very limited effect on gingival contour and on the access to *visible* tooth surfaces for self-performed plaque control. Surgery is not, therefore, performed in order to *create* good gingival contours.

However, it is important to employ a technique of surgery which will allow the *re-establishment* of favourable gingival contours during healing.

The ultimate aim of periodontal therapy must be the regeneration of predisease quantities of healthy periodontium. However, at present, there are great practical difficulties in achieving this (*see* Chapter 20). We are, therefore, obliged to accept as a realistic aim the restoration to health of remaining periodontal support, i.e. the arrest, but not reversal, of connective tissue attachment loss.

Surgery is indicated after a phase of hygiene therapy for residual deep pathological pockets at sites where plaque control is good.

Careful reference to the treatment planning chart is necessary. If hygiene therapy has been properly carried out and good oral hygiene has been established, there will be no *shallow* pathological pockets since these will have been instrumented adequately. Residual pathological pockets will be those where access for non-surgical instrumentation was poor and these pockets will be relatively deep.

In considering the desired level of oral hygiene, the practice of setting a threshold value for supragingival plaque-infected surfaces (commonly 5–15% of all tooth surfaces in the mouth), below which surgical intervention may be considered, is not a good one. It is well established that the same tooth surfaces consistently remain cleaned or not cleaned irrespective of the overall level of performance. Surgical intervention, therefore, *would* be justified, say, for clean incisors even when plaque is present throughout most of the rest of the dentition. Conversely, the only residual pathological pockets following hygiene therapy may lie within the one small area of the dentition where the patient's plaque control capabilities are poor. Surgery at these sites would not be successful and should *not* be attempted unless there is good reason to believe that plaque control will be better after surgery; for example, patients who find flossing difficult may accomplish interdental cleaning quite effectively after surgery if sufficient interdental space has been created to accommodate an interdental brush.

Where doubt exists concerning the adeqacy of plaque control, surgery may be carried out for a single segment of the dentition and further surgery postponed until the adequacy of postoperative plaque control can be confirmed.

Surgical techniques for the treatment of periodontitis are sometimes differentiated by the priority given to pocket elimination or reattachment. The main differences are in the management of bone and method of wound closure; the main objective in each case is a physiological gingival sulcus. During 'pocket elimination', the soft tissue forming the pocket wall is resected or repositioned apically with formation, during healing, of a new gingival margin at a more apical level. Bony pocket walls are also resected. 'Reattachment' requires the preservation of gingival soft tissue with formation of a long epithelial attachment to the planed root surface. Often elements of both reattachment and pocket elimination are combined.

In this textbook, the technique recommended for anterior and premolar regions is 'open-flap curettage', a reattachment procedure. Pocket elimination is advocated for the surgical management of molar periodontitis. A description of each technique follows.

Open-flap Curettage

Several longitudinal clinical studies (e.g. Rosling *et al.*, 1976*b*; Knowles *et al.*, 1980) have shown that the best technique in most areas of the dentition is one in which flaps are raised with minimal sacrifice of soft tissue to give access for root instrumentation, then replaced at or close to their presurgical position to form an epithelial attachment to the tooth surface. This replaced flap procedure is sometimes referred to as an 'access flap', 'flap surgery for reattachment', a 'modified Widman flap' or, perhaps more logically, as 'open-flap curettage'. This approach to surgical treatment was popularised by Ramfjord and Nissle (1974) and Ramfjord (1977) who coined the expression 'modified Widman flap'. Many minor variations of this technique exist. The method about to be described differs from Ramfjord's original description principally with respect to the incisions employed.

a)   An intracrevicular incision is made around the necks of the teeth buccally, lingually and interproximally (Fig. 10.2(a)). If a deep pocket is present at one end of the marginal incision, a vertical relieving incision may be required on the buccal aspect to provide proper access. This is preferable to the risk of tearing the flap as a result of stretching it to gain access, and probably also preferable to extending the

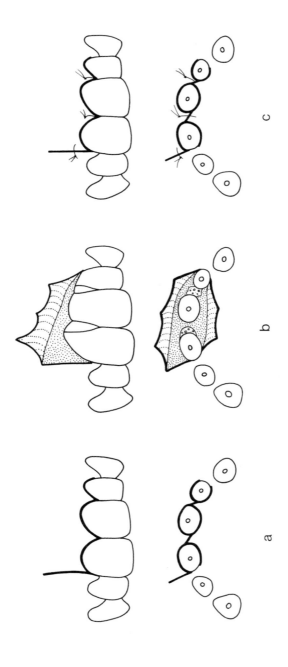

Fig. 10.2 *Open-flap curettage. (a) Marginal intracrevicular and vertical relieving incisions; (b) buccal and palatal mucoperiosteal flaps reflected to expose marginal bone and interdental bone defects; (c) wound closure with simple interrupted sutures.*

marginal incision beyond the diseased area, which would be an alternative method of improving access. Vertical incisions are unnecessary on lingual or palatal aspects.

The intracrevicular marginal incision is a departure from the more traditional inverse or reverse bevel incision (Fig. 10.3). The latter was designed to excise the pocket lining containing epithelium and infiltrated connective tissue in the belief, no longer held, that new connective tissue attachment to the root surface might thereby occur. A number of studies have shown that the intracrevicular incision gives as good results as the reverse bevel incision (Svoboda *et al.*, 1984; Lindhe and Nyman, 1985; Smith *et al.*, 1987). Moreover, since none of the marginal gingiva is sacrificed, there can be no difficulty in achieving flap closure.

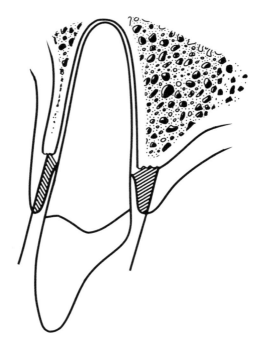

Fig. 10.3   *Reverse-bevel incisions for flap procedures. The shaded areas are excised.*

b) Full-thickness mucoperiosteal flaps are elevated on both buccal and lingual/palatal aspects to expose the marginal bone (Fig. 10.2(b)).

c) Granulation tissue adhering to the bone is removed and the roots are scaled and planed until hard and smooth.

d) The repair potential of tissues affected by periodontitis must be fully exploited in order to restore or at least preserve periodontal support, avoid increased tooth mobility and maintain gingival height. Bone contouring, therefore, should be avoided but may occasionally be necessary to facilitate root planing or flap closure. There is nothing to be gained by trying to make bony contours conform to some imagined 'physiological' ideal. This could result in loss of support to adjacent unaffected tooth surfaces. In any case, many defects, particularly those with three bone walls, possess good potential for bone-fill.

e) The flaps are replaced with interrupted sutures (Fig. 10.2(c)). Periodontal dressing is unnecessary since complete wound closure should have been achieved. Chlorhexidine mouthwash is prescribed so that the wound will be saved from the physical trauma of tooth cleaning and so that the patient will be spared the discomfort of cleaning tender gingivae and sensitive root surfaces.

f) Sutures are removed one week later.

Healing after Open-flap Curettage

When close adaptation of buccal and lingual flap margins is achieved following open-flap curettage, healing by primary intention may occur. Sometimes, however, the tissue contraction associated with wound healing prevents the union of buccal and lingual flap margins and a soft-tissue interdental crater is produced.

When an intracrevicular incision has been employed, the pocket epithelium, which has been replaced against the root surface, undergoes involution and forms junctional epithelium. A mature epithelial attachment forms in two to four weeks.

When infrabony lesions are present, bony repair may occur within the boundaries of the bone defect, usually accompanied by some crestal resorption. However, there will be a strand of junctional epithelium interposed between the regenerated bone tissue and the root surface.

Advantages of Open-flap Curettage

a)   Postoperative recession is minimised, giving optimum aesthetics, minimal exposure of sensitive dentine and minimal risk of root caries and speech impairment.

b)   Rapid healing is achieved with minimal postoperative discomfort and periodontal dressing is usually unnecessary. With no exposed areas to granulate and epithelialise, patients are soon able to resume mechanical plaque control instead of relying on chlorhexidine for a lengthy period with its inconvenient side-effects.

c)   Supporting bone can be retained and optimal bone-fill within infrabony pockets should be achieved. The occlusal stability conferred by good bony support is very advantageous towards the front of the mouth, where tooth migration is particularly undesirable.

d)   Longitudinal studies have shown that, in the treatment of deep pockets, this technique leads to a greater gain of clinical attachment than that obtainable by any other surgical method in routine use.

Disadvantages of Open-flap Curettage

a)   Thorough scaling and root planing at the time of surgery is mandatory when reattachment is desired. Failure to achieve this through inadequate surgical exposure will negate any advantage in the technique. In this respect, good access for adequate root instrumentation in molar regions is often difficult to achieve.

b)   The close interdental apposition of buccal and lingual flap margins is an important facet of this technique. However, flap margins frequently fail to unite and wound contraction may produce an interdental soft-tissue crater. Regeneration of interdental tissues will tend to occur but this may take several months and, if the crater is deep enough to inhibit interdental cleaning, inflammation will recur. Gingivoplasty, to remove one or both crater margins, may be necessary once it becomes apparent that natural remodelling is going to be inadequate. This is inconvenient but cannot be considered a major disadvantage.

c)   Open-flap curettage is generally a less suitable technique for use between molars: the much broader proximal contact surfaces of these teeth prevent the interdental gingiva from

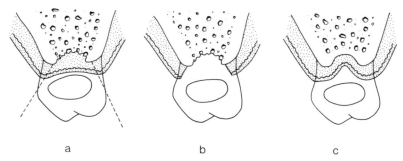

a   b   c

Fig. 10.4 *Open-flap curettage for molar teeth. Section through interdental space with proximal contact surface outlined. (a) Marginal incisions are made (broken line); (b) owing to loss of interdental gingiva, wound closure cannot be achieved; (c) during healing, interdental soft tissue conforms to underlying bone contour.*

being readily removed, attached to one or other of the buccal or lingual flaps (Fig. 10.4). Instead, the interdental gingiva usually has to be sacrificed and close apposition of buccal and lingual flap margins often cannot be achieved at the end of the operation. If a bone defect is present, this will granulate from its base, new gingival tissue will conform to the underlying bone contour and result in a particularly deep soft-tissue interdental crater. Interdental cleaning is difficult enough in molar regions without the added complication of gingival deformity. An alternative surgical approach for molar periodontitis is, therefore, described below.

d)   Where a restoration extends into a periodontal pocket, there is little point in covering this restoration with soft tissue at the end of the operation. Although, in theory, 'reattachment' to clean restoration surfaces may occur, in practice bacterial residues at the tooth–restoration interface are likely to re-create a pathological pocket. Open-flap curettage should not, therefore, be carried out for restorations which extend more than 0·5 mm beyond the gingival margin. Instead, sufficient gingival tissue should be excised to locate the restoration supragingivally at the end of the operation. Another way of dealing with the soft tissue rather than excising some of it, is to reposition the flap apically, and this is to be preferred in areas of narrow gingival width. If the restoration extends to within approximately 4 mm of the alveolar crest, bone would also have to be removed to leave room for postoperative gingival regrowth (*see* Chapter 17).

Pocket Elimination for Molar Periodontitis

In molar regions, the use of a pocket-elimination technique, rather than a reattachment technique, is necessitated by the lack of sufficient soft tissue for proper wound closure. Figure 10.4 illustrates the likely outcome if open-flap curettage is attempted. The recommended approach is as follows.

a)   Intracrevicular or reverse-bevel incisions are made in the usual way (Fig. 10.5(a)) and buccal and lingual/palatal

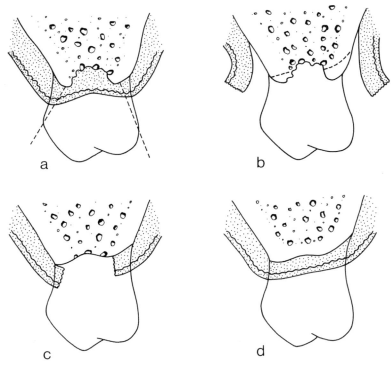

Fig. 10.5   *Pocket elimination for molar periodontitis. (a) Marginal incisions. (b) Buccal and palatal flaps reflected; broken line indicates extent of planned osteoplasty. (c) Flaps replaced after osteoplasty. (d) Interdental gingival contour after healing of exposed interdental bone.*

mucoperiosteal flaps are elevated to expose the affected root surfaces (Fig. 10.5(b)).

b) Granulation tissue is removed and the root surfaces are curetted.

c) The interdental bone should be inspected for defects. If none exist, then wound closure should proceed as described in (d) below. If a three-wall bone defect is present, this should be allowed to fill with a blood clot since good potential will exist for bone regeneration even though the defect cannot be covered by soft tissue. In this situation, a long junctional epithelium is interposed between the new bone and the tooth surface, providing an element of reattachment in what is otherwise a pocket-elimination technique. Usually an interdental bone crater will be present which will have to be recontoured to allow the establishment of a satisfactory interdental soft-tissue contour during healing. This recontouring may be carried out as illustrated in Figure 10.5(b) and (c). Other types of bone defect may be found and may also need to be reshaped. This will mean removal of supporting bone from the less affected tooth and should be kept to the minimum necessary to achieve an adequate contour. Fortunately, such bone defects often have more walls apically than at the bone crest so that the healing potential of the three walls can often be exploited by eliminating only the coronal portion of the defect.

d) The flaps should be readapted around the necks of the teeth and the relationships of the flaps to the underlying bone should be assessed before suturing. If the flap margins are thin and, on the buccal aspect, there is adequate attached gingiva and vestibular depth, interdental sutures can be placed without further adjustment (Fig. 10.5(c)). Frequently, however, the palatal flap has a thick fibrous margin, not readily adaptable to the underlying bone (Fig. 10.6(a)). Because it is not possible to reposition a palatal flap in an apical direction, the flap margin must instead be thinned either by papillectomy (Fig. 10.6(b)) or by an undermining incision. In the lower arch, a similar approach may be necessary to deal with thick fibrous lingual flaps. A further possible complication is depicted in Figure 10.7(a) where there is a narrow zone of buccal gingiva and the corrected bone margin is close to the vestibular fornix. If the buccal and palatal flaps were sutured tightly together, the small

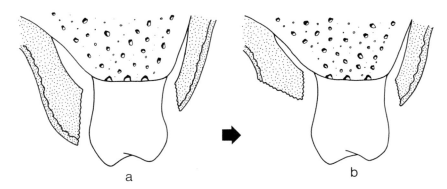

Fig. 10.6   *Pocket elimination for molar periodontitis; management of thickened palatal flap margin. (a) Osteoplasty has been carried out. (b) Palatal gingivectomy to allow better flap adaptation to tooth and bone.*

amount of buccal gingiva would be pulled into the interdental space and the vestibule would be obliterated. The buccal flap should, therefore, be repositioned apically, thereby deepening the vestibule and maintaining an 'adequate' zone of attached gingiva (Fig. 10.7(b)). Apical repositioning can be achieved by inserting simple interrupted interdental sutures, the tensions of which are adjusted so that the flap will be displaced apically to the desired position by the periodontal dressing.

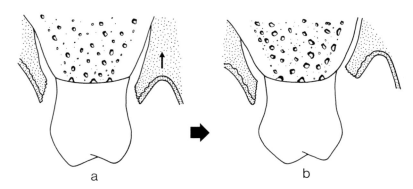

Fig. 10.7   *Pocket elimination for molar periodontitis: apical repositioning. (a) Osteoplasty has been carried out with loss of vestibular depth; small arrow indicates planned apical displacement of buccal flap. (b) Location of flap margins before suturing.*

e)   After the placement of interdental sutures, the wound is protected by periodontal dressing.

f)   The periodontal dressing and sutures are removed one week later, by which time interdental granulation tissue will have formed and epithelialisation will have commenced. Occasionally, it may be necessary to apply a fresh periodontal dressing for one further week.

Healing after Pocket-elimination Flap Surgery

Where interdental soft-tissue coverage has not been achieved between molars, granulation tissue proliferates from the flap margins, periodontal membrane and exposed bone. Simultaneously, epithelial cells proliferate at the flap margins and migrate across the wound. Soft-tissue maturation proceeds with some coronal regrowth of tissue and the formation of a new epithelial attachment. In areas where the flaps were laid against the tooth surface, healing proceeds as described for the open-flap curettage procedure. Thus, using the technique described above, a new marginal gingiva and dentogingival junction of normal dimensions is created at a more apical level, close to the base of the original pocket (Fig. 10.5(d)). Narrowly defined, the term 'pocket elimination' will apply only when both the soft tissue and bony walls of the pocket have been eliminated. However, three-wall infrabony pockets are usually left to granulate in the expectation that bone-fill will occur, in spite of the absence of flap coverage.

Advantages of Pocket Elimination

a)   A dentoepithelial junction of normal dimensions is produced. In the event of recurrent periodontitis, the pockets arising should be shallow and further treatment will be simplified.

b)   Interdental spaces are enlarged. This may improve access for plaque control.

c)   Restoration margins which were formerly subgingival may become supragingival following surgery. The existence of pathological pockets occupied by subgingival restorations is an important indication for pocket elimination, rather than open-flap curettage.

d)   Pocket elimination does not depend to a very great extent on the ability of the operator to carry out extensive scaling and root planing at the time of surgery. This is because much of the affected root surface will be exposed in the mouth postoperatively and will not be required to accommodate healing gingival tissue. Poor access in posterior regions is, therefore, an indication for pocket elimination.

Disadvantages of Pocket Elimination

a)   Large areas of dentine may be exposed with risk of hypersensitivity. Plaque control may suffer and the risk of relapse and caries will increase.

b)   Supporting bone may have to be removed to eliminate an infrabony pocket. This may be quite impracticable in the case of a deep infrabony pocket and a compromise solution is, therefore, required.

c)   Exposed root anatomy such as proximal concavities may complicate plaque control.

d)   The technique of pocket elimination is described in this text for use only in molar regions. It is not aesthetically acceptable in anterior or premolar regions, particularly in the upper arch.

PLANNING OF PERIODONTAL SURGERY

It should be ascertained that all teeth for which surgery may be desirable, are accessible both for surgery and subsequent home care. In this respect, upper second and third molars may be particularly awkward because of the proximity of the coronoid process of the mandible when the mouth is open. There may be a small oral aperture, narrow arches or a hyperactive tongue as well as peculiarities of tooth position.

Surgery may be carried out in segments, quadrants, arches, half or whole mouths according to circumstances. For example, complex techniques, such as those which may be required to manage furcation lesions, should generally be restricted to one segment. Although the patient may be less inconvenienced by a surgical programme condensed into one or two extended appointments, it is the clinician's responsibility to ensure that he does not attempt too much at one sitting, so that the procedure may be completed satisfactorily without leaving clinician or patient physically or emotionally drained. The tolerance of the patient and finesse of the operator may be stretched if periodontal surgical procedures are extended beyond 45–60 minutes.

Informed consent should be sought and this will entail advising the patient of the reasons for surgery, the need for continued plaque control, the nature, number and duration of procedures and their anticipated side-effects, such as discomfort, swelling and gingival recession.

SURGICAL PRINCIPLES

Local anaesthesia should commence whenever possible by block injection to minimise the number of injections. Teeth, as well as periodontium, should be anaesthetised to avoid eliciting pain during scaling and root planing. When anaesthesia has been achieved, papillary infiltration is employed to reduce blood loss and improve visibility.

Management of Soft Tissue

Following initial incisions for flap procedures, full-thickness (mucoperiosteal) flaps are raised by blunt dissection. The flap should be raised only as far as is necessary to gain access or achieve any desired repositioning. Gauze sponges moistened with saline may be used at various stages during surgery to contain haemorrhage within interdental spaces. Removal of granulation tissue will further reduce haemorrhage and facilitate inspection of bone margins and root furcations. It is often only at this stage that final decisions can be taken about bone recontouring and flap closure.

Management of Bone

When bone removal is necessary, recontouring should be carried out as atraumatically as possible using appropriately shaped burs or coarse-bonded stones rotating slowly with adequate saline irrigation or using hand-held chisels or files. Thorough irrigation should follow recontouring to ensure that all debris is removed from the wound.

Management of Tooth Substance

The recontouring of tooth substance is undertaken most frequently in relation to early furcation involvement and this will be dealt with in Chapter 11. However, on occasion, it will be desirable to reduce the groove sometimes found on the palatal aspect of upper incisors or the root concavity or fossa of posterior teeth, notably the upper first premolar. This should be carried out judiciously, bearing in mind the risk of postoperative dentine sensitivity and caries.

COMPARISON OF TECHNIQUES

It is of fundamental importance that details of surgical techniques are not allowed to obscure the prerequisites for successful surgical pocket therapy, namely adequate débridement at operation and adequate plaque control subsequently. The reader is urged to recognise that there are, nevertheless, advantages and disadvantages in each technique. The reader should review the work of Zamet (1975), Rosling *et al.* (1976*a*), Nyman *et al.* (1977) and Knowles *et al.* (1980). The conclusions of Rosling (1976*b*), regarding patients maintained on an optimal level of oral hygiene, may be summarised as follows.

a) Healthy gingival conditions can be achieved and maintained, irrespective of surgical technique.
b) Periodontal disease can be cured and the continuous progression of destructive marginal periodontitis terminated, irrespective of surgical technique.
c) Different techniques of surgical pocket therapy will allow the periodontal tissues to heal but may promote varying degrees of tissue reorganisation.
d) The largest amount of bone-fill within angular bony defects is obtained not only when resection of bone is avoided but when, in addition, the alveolar bone is completely covered by the mucoperiosteal flaps.

PROBLEM AREAS

The management of certain special areas of a dentition must be planned in conjunction with flap surgery. Such areas include tooth surfaces adjacent to edentulous areas, the retromolar and tuberosity regions, furcation lesions, combined periodontal–pulpal lesions and unerupted teeth. While basic principles still apply, the surgical management of edentulous and retromolar areas can be difficult. On the other hand, access to tooth surfaces adjacent to such areas may be adequate for scaling without surgical access. A number of techniques for surgery have been described and these are covered in the standard textbooks. The management of furcation and combined periodontal–pulpal lesions will be described in Chapters 11 and 12.

The management of third molar teeth is worthy of further consideration. The third molar should be evaluated from two standpoints: association with pathology and likely usefulness.

The fully erupted tooth should be assessed with regard to position and function, possibly as an abutment, and feasibility of maintaining satisfactory oral hygiene. The interdental area between second and third molars may be difficult to clean and it may be unrealistic to try to maintain both teeth. Careful assessment of crown and periodontium including furcation examination and vitality tests, if indicated, should be made before condemning either tooth.

The same arguments may be applied to partially erupted teeth in good position to erupt normally. These teeth may be affected by pericoronitis and one must try to assess the likelihood of this being recurrent. The treatment of recurrent pericoronitis is likely to be removal of the third molar during a quiescent phase but, occasionally, removal of the second molar will allow the third molar to erupt into good position. However, this is a hazardous approach and should usually be reserved for circumstances in which the second molar cannot be maintained or has a very poor prognosis.

Unerupted and impacted teeth may be associated with follicular enlargement, root resorption or chronic infection via sinus or periodontal pocket, all of which may prejudice the periodontal support of the distal root of the second molar. The aims of periodontal surgery in relation to the second molar may be impossible to fulfil as long as an unerupted or impacted third molar is present. It will usually be advisable, therefore, to remove it either at the time of periodontal surgery or in advance. Failure to do this may lead to an unstable or unpredictable periodontal condition. Finally, the opportunity of autotransplantation should be considered for the very rare occasions when a first molar must be removed and an unerupted third molar of similar morphology can be atraumatically transplanted.

POSTOPERATIVE CARE

Complications of periodontal surgery are unusual, but postoperative bleeding may occur unexpectedly. This is usually easily controlled if the bleeding area is identified and pressure applied. Rinsing, heat and alcohol should be avoided and the patient should be in a sitting position.

Postoperative pain and swelling are usually mild and transient. Both are loosely related to the duration of the procedure and extent to which tissues are traumatised, but pain is also a function of attitude and personality. Acute or pyogenic wound infection is rare but may occur if debris is left beneath the flap.

If is of fundamental importance that operated tooth surfaces do not become plaque-infected during healing or indeed subsequently. To this end, patients must be given detailed instruction in the home care of operated and adjacent areas in the postoperative period and be seen frequently enough to ensure that such instructions are carried out and that they are effective. Mechanical cleaning must generally be abandoned in the operated area for the first two weeks after surgery, because of the presence of either periodontal dressing or discomfort and should be replaced by a regime of rinsing with 0·2% chlorhexidine— 10 ml for two minutes twice daily at normal tooth cleaning times. This regime should be continued until the patient can clean mechanically without bleeding or discomfort.

When, in spite of efforts to avoid it at the time of surgery, a soft-tissue crater develops postoperatively, the use of chlorhexidine may have to be continued for a few weeks. With meticulous plaque control, gingiva will tend to seek a scalloped contour which will facilitate subsequent mechanical plaque control measures. If plaque infection of root surfaces is allowed to occur, either epithelial attachment will not take place and a pocket will result, or gingival regeneration will be suppressed.

With the reinstitution of mechanical cleaning, oral hygiene measures should be reappraised in the light of the new gingival contour. Frequently, interdental brushes can be substituted for dental floss and this should be encouraged where possible as most patients find interdental brushes easier to use.

Postoperative Sequelae

These should be anticipated and patients advised accordingly.

Tooth mobility frequently increases after periodontal surgery and may not peak until three weeks after surgery. It will then fall over three to six months to preoperative levels or less, provided supporting bone has not been removed. Teeth associated with infrabony defects and mobile before surgery may be stabilised by bone-fill of such defects.

Dentine hypersensitivity may be a problem, as large areas of newly planed root surface may be exposed to chemical, thermal and mechanical stimuli in the mouth. This may be severe enough to preclude adequate tooth cleaning and may reflect a transient pulpal hyperaemia due to the instrumentation of the root surface. Thermal stimuli will be more noticeable because of the loss of the insulating layer of gingival soft tissue.

Many 'desensitising' agents are available but the rationale for their use is still somewhat obscure. Nevertheless, patients do report improvement following application of fluoride preparations such as gels and varnishes which will also provide some protection against root surface caries. Dentine hypersensitivity should be treated aggressively in order to avoid the risk of recurrent periodontal disease as a result of plaque accumulation in sensitive areas.

Periodontal surgery may expose to carious attack a number of new sites in a mouth with little recent caries experience. One must be alert to the possibility of renewed caries activity. Satisfactory results will be achieved and untoward sequelae avoided only if a regime of close supervision for reinforcement of oral hygiene is adopted. Patients should be seen frequently until the clinician is satisfied that adequate oral hygiene is being maintained, when the interval between recall visits may be gradually extended (*see* Chapter 16).

REFERENCES

Knowles J., Burgett F., Morrison E., Nissle R., Ramfjord S. (1980). Comparison of results following three modalities of periodontal therapy related to tooth type and initial pocket depth. *Journal of Clinical Periodontology*; 7: 32–47.

Lindhe J., Nyman S. (1985). Scaling and granulation tissue removal in periodontal therapy. *Journal of Clinical Periodontology*; 12: 374–88.

Nyman S., Lindhe J., Rosling B. (1977). Periodontal surgery in plaque-infected dentitions. *Journal of Clinical Periodontology*; 4: 240–9.

Ramfjord S.P., Nissle R. R. (1974). The modified Widman flap. *Journal of Periodontology*; 45: 601–7.

Ramfjord S. P. (1977). Present status of the modified Widman flap procedure. *Journal of Periodontology*; 48: 558–65.

Rosling B., Nyman S., Lindhe J. (1976*a*). The effect of systematic plaque control on bone regeneration in infra-bony pockets. *Journal of Clinical Periodontology*; 3: 38–53.

Rosling B., Nyman S., Lindhe J., Jern B. (1976*b*). The healing potential of the periodontal tissues following different techniques of periodontal surgery in plaque-free dentitions. *Journal of Clinical Periodontology*; 3: 233–50.

Smith B. A., Echeverri M., Caffesse R. G. (1987). Mucoperiosteal flaps with and without removal of pocket epithelium. *Journal of Periodontology*; 58: 78–85.

Svoboda P. J., Reeve C. M., Sheridan P. J. (1984). Effect of retention of gingival sulcular epithelium on attachment and pocket depth after periodontal surgery. *Journal of Periodontology*; 55: 563–6.

Zamet J. S. (1975). A comparative clinical study of three periodontal surgical techniques. *Journal of Clinical Periodontology*; 2: 87–97.

FURTHER READING

Barrington E. P. (1981). An overview of periodontal surgical procedures. *Journal of Periodontology*; 52: 518–28.

Kakehashi S., Parakkal P. E. (1982). Surgical therapy for periodontitis. *Journal of Periodontology*; 53: 477–501.

Ramfjord S. P., Knowles J., Nissle R., Burgett F., Shick R. (1975). Results following three modalities of periodontal therapy. *Journal of Periodontology*; 46: 522–6.

Waite I. M. (1975). Present status of gingivectomy procedure. *Journal of Clinical Periodontology*; 2: 241–9.

Wirthlin M. R. (1981). Current status of new attachment therapy. *Journal of Periodontology*; 52: 529–44.

Chapter 11

Management of Furcation Lesions

DEFINITION

The furcation lesion (furcation involvement) is an extension of periodontitis with connective tissue attachment loss between the roots of multirooted teeth, typically the molars and upper first premolars. However, other teeth may exhibit aberrations of root anatomy and may develop furcation lesions. The only peculiarity of the lesion is its anatomical situation. In all respects the lesion is similar to that on a single-rooted tooth except that, during invasion of the furcation area, connective tissue attachment loss and epithelial migration on the root surface take place horizontally as well as vertically. It is the inaccessibility of the lesion which necessitates special mention. Pulp pathology may also give rise to furcation lesions and this will be discussed in Chapter 12.

CLASSIFICATION

There is wide acceptance of three classes of furcation lesion.

Grade I—incipient or shallow cave. This is the earliest stage in the development of the lesion, sometimes said to extend up to 3 mm of *horizontal* connective tissue loss.
Grade II—partial or deep cave, between incipient and through-and-through.
Grade III—through-and-through involvement which extends from one furcation entrance to another.

While this classification is useful for descriptive purposes, it is only of limited value in treatment planning.

AETIOLOGY

The primary aetiological factor is accumulation of bacterial plaque. This is enhanced by various predisposing factors, the most significant of which is the local anatomy and root morphology.

Anatomy

The majority of multirooted teeth are situated in posterior regions of the mouth. This presents obvious difficulties of access for both treatment and home care.

Posterior teeth have broader contact areas than anterior teeth and so are even less amenable to adequate plaque control by the toothbrush alone. This, in turn, increases the likelihood of caries of approximal surfaces and the need for restoration of these surfaces which, in the case of upper posterior teeth, are adjacent to the mesial and distal furcations. Restoration and tooth cleaning may be further complicated by approximal surface root concavities. These may harbour plaque and calculus or create difficulty in adaptation of matrix bands.

A peculiarity of cervical tooth anatomy is the 'enamel projection'. This is an apical projection of enamel towards the furcation, most commonly of buccal surfaces, and may lead to early furcation involvement by allowing rapid apical growth of plaque and spread of inflammation.

It is essential to acknowledge the scope for variation in root morphology. Approximately 50% of upper first premolars have two roots. The majority of upper first molars have three roots and three furcations, mesial, distal and buccal, and most lower first molars have a mesial and distal root and so buccal and lingual furcations. Second and third molars are less predictable and exhibit more variations of this basic pattern. Length, curvature and divergence of roots vary widely, as does the distance apical to the amelocemental junction at which the furcation begins. This distance may be different for each furcation of the same tooth and, indeed, any individual furcation may be absent because of fusion of adjacent roots. Roots which are distinctly separate coronally may be fused apically. One should be aware also of the possibility of rarer variations such as three-rooted lower canines!

The upper first molar will bear further elaboration (Fig. 11.1). The mesiobuccal root, though often narrow mesiodistally (as seen on radiography), is normally broad buccopalatally and so the mesial furcation tends to be situated palatally. The palatal root tends to be sturdy, straight and round in cross-section, but

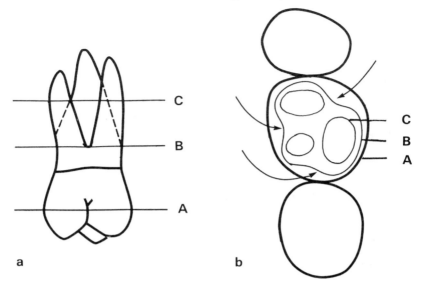

Fig. 11.1 *The upper molar trifurcation.* (a) *Upper first molar seen from the buccal aspect showing three planes of section A, B, C.* (b) *Cross section through upper first molar showing levels A, B, C (superimposed). Level A illustrates the relationship of the crown to adjacent teeth. Level B shows the entrances to the trifurcation (arrowed). Level C indicates the relative size and position of the three roots.*

frequently diverges from the long axis of the tooth and may be affected by recession. It tends to be situated distally. The foregoing indicates that the mesial furcation will be more readily examined from the palatal aspect (Fig. 11.2). The distal root is usually the smallest in cross-section and length. The distal furcation tends to be beneath the marginal ridge and situated slightly towards the buccal owing to the greater diameter of the palatal root, and so the distal furcation is usually examined from the buccal side. Finally, because of the small circumference of the distobuccal root, other things being equal, Grade III furcation involvement is likely to occur first between the buccal and distal furcations.

Iatrogenic Factors

The furcation lesion is an extension of an initial marginal lesion. Marginal bone loss is acknowledged to be more common

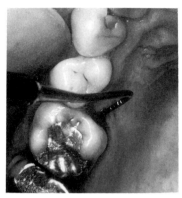

Fig. 11.2 *Williams periodontal probe in the mesial furcation of an upper first molar. Note how far palatally the furcation is situated owing to the breadth of the mesiobuccal root.*

adjacent to overhanging margins of restorations. Approximal surfaces of posterior teeth are susceptible to caries and late diagnosis will result in large restorations which are more likely to have overhanging margins, especially if matrix bands are used without adequate wedging. It follows, then, that early diagnosis of caries is important and that matrices should be wedged and a check made for overhangs which should be removed during carving. Finally, the restored surface should be checked for cervical fit using dental floss and a fine probe. Crown margins should also be checked in this way.

Occlusion

The contribution which occlusal forces might make to the progression of periodontal disease has been discussed in Chapter 4. There is no reason to believe that occlusal forces contribute to the development of furcation lesions. Mobility is a late sign of furcation involvement and, according to Waerhaug (1980), is not involved in its aetiology. This late development of mobility is probably one reason for late diagnosis, when treatment may be difficult or impossible.

OCCURRENCE AND DISTRIBUTION

The distribution of teeth with furcated root morphology has already been described. The occurrence of furcation lesions will rise with increasing severity of periodontal disease. This tends to be greatest interdentally, and so mesial and distal furcations (upper molars and premolars) are more vulnerable than lingual or buccal furcations, where periodontal disease progresses more slowly. The upper first molar, when present, is the tooth most likely to be affected by a furcation lesion, since periodontal disease tends to be more advanced at first molar sites than elsewhere and their roots tend to separate more coronally than do those of second and third molars.

Ross and Thomson (1980) have reported furcation lesions in 90% of upper molars and 35% of lower molars in a population of periodontal patients.

DIAGNOSIS

Furcation lesions can be diagnosed by careful clinical examination using the periodontal probe or gently curved instruments such as curettes, which may be introduced horizontally to the mesial and distal furcations. It should be possible to feel the roof of the furcation in this way, so confirming its involvement. The full extent of furcation involvement may be difficult to evaluate clinically without resort to surgical exploration (Hamp *et al.*, 1975). Radiographic examination, possibly using the parallax technique, may reveal additional detail. However, because of the superimposition of roots in the upper premolar and molar areas the extent of involvement can easily be underestimated, and so radiographs should not be relied upon.

The clinical and radiographic examination must also reveal whether the tooth can be restored to function. This will entail assessment of the occlusion, the feasibility of restoring the crown, the status of the pulp, gingival condition, root canal anatomy and the need to replace any missing teeth.

TREATMENT

The general principles of treatment planning outlined in Chapter 7 can be applied to management of teeth with furcation lesions. The treatment options can be related to the degree of involvement. However, one must also consider the patient's age and predisposition to periodontal disease, motivation and manual dexterity in plaque control. In planning treatment one must try to assess the likelihood of tooth survival with various treatment options. This may be relatively easy with single-rooted teeth, but multirooted teeth are more likely to be affected by acute infection or endodontic involvement via lateral or accessory canals, which are said to be common in furcations.

The following protocol describes the treatment options for each grade of furcation lesion in the order in which each option should be considered.

Grade I
   a)   Scaling and root planing.
   b)   Surgical pocket therapy.
   c)   Furcation-plasty.
   d)   Root resection (rarely).

Grade II
   a)   Scaling and root planing in conjunction with surgical pocket therapy.
   b)   Root resection.
   c)   'Maintenance' with hygiene therapy alone.
   d)   Extraction.

Grade III
   a)   Scaling and root planing with surgical pocket therapy and root resection.
   b)   Tunnel preparation.
   c)   'Maintenance' with hygiene therapy.
   d)   Extraction.

In patients with a complete dentition where all molars have furcation involvement, a treatment plan aiming to restore all the molars to periodontal health is seldom rational. Such treatment is likely to be too extensive in relation to the expected benefits and might preserve a dentition too complicated for satisfactory plaque control (Nyman and Lindhe, 1976). It is not possible to provide general rules about which teeth should be maintained or extracted. One must try to select which teeth may be most simply restored to function with good prognosis. Thus, one must consider the feasibility of satisfactory treatment. Is access sufficient for scaling, surgery and home care? Is endodontic treatment required in conjunction with root separation techniques and are the root morphology and root canal anatomy favourable? Can the crowns be restored?

Scaling and Root Planing

Scaling and root planing may be carried out without surgical access or as part of surgical pocket therapy if better access is required for thorough débridement. These measures will often be sufficient for Grade I lesions but success is less predictable in Grade II lesions where these measures are often no more than palliative.

Furcation-plasty

This entails recontouring tooth and/or bone to create a shallow vertical groove, from the bone apical to the furcation through the site of the lesion and coronally to approximately half the height of the crown. Access is thus permitted for completion of scaling and root planing and creation of a dental and gingival contour which can be readily maintained plaque-free (Fig. 11.3). Extensive furcation-plasty may predispose to dentine hypersensitivity and caries. Furcation-plasty may be readily applied to buccal and lingual furcations but is less often feasible on mesial and distal surfaces. Adequate treatment of these lesions may necessitate root resection.

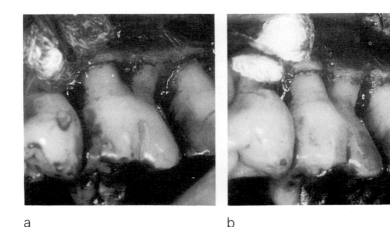

a   b

Fig. 11.3 *Furcation-plasty. (a) Flap elevated to expose a buccal furcation lesion on /6. (b) Furcation-plasty has been carried out. Note the change in contour of marginal bone and adjacent tooth surface.*

Root Resection

Many Grade II or III furcation lesions are inaccessible for scaling and root planing even with surgical access and, therefore, their certain elimination can be achieved only by root resection. However, the necessity for root canal therapy beforehand and often crown restoration afterwards must be considered and, where these resources are limited, an alternative approach to treatment may need to be sought. Root resection, nevertheless, should be attempted in carefully selected patients where patient cooperation is not in doubt, the prognosis for the dentition is good and execution of treatment is likely to be straightforward. The following considerations should, then, be kept in mind.

a) It is desirable, but not essential, that the roots to be retained are endodontically treated before separation. It is helpful if the coronal third of the root canal and the portion of the pulp chamber to be sectioned are filled with amalgam prior to sectioning, as this obviates the need to seal the sectioned surface at the time of surgery. Roots which are retained to be restored with post-retained crowns or as bridge abutments should not have their root canals obturated in this way.

b) Sometimes a definite decision about which root or roots to retain can be made only after surgical exploration or division of the crown and roots, to allow assessment of mobility and probing of the furcation surfaces of the roots. In such circumstances of doubtful prognosis, endodontic treatment may be delayed until after surgery. An effort should be made to retain sufficient tooth substance to facilitate application of a rubber dam.

c) Prognosis will depend on satisfactory endodontic *and* periodontal treatment.

d) The mobility of individual roots after separation will exceed the mobility of the whole tooth.

e) With regard to lower molars, the mesial root usually has two pulp canals, the distal only one. Moreover, access to the distal canal may be easier, owing to mesial angulation.

f) With regard to upper molars, morphology is variable but generally the mesiobuccal root is the most useful, being broad buccopalatally and in the line of the arch. However, some 60% may have two root canals. The palatal root may be difficult to restore to function because of its tendency to

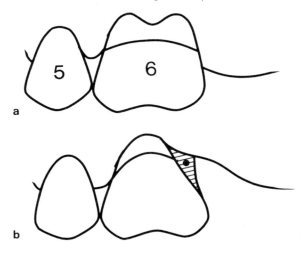

Fig. 11.4 *Crown contour* (a) *before and* (b) *after resection of distobuccal root of upper left first molar.*

diverge from the long axis of the tooth. The distobuccal root is small and rarely retained alone. The crown of the upper first molar may be readily retained intact following removal of the distobuccal root alone. (Fig. 11.4). Minor recontouring will leave a form which can be more readily maintained than if either the mesiobuccal or palatal root alone is removed.

g)   Root resection is not a worthwhile option for upper first premolars.

Buccal and lingual flaps should always be raised, and the process of sectioning should start in the affected furcation. It may be possible to insert a probe into the opposite furcation entrance to indicate the direction of cut to be made. The cut should be made with a sharp bur or diamond stone under copious saline irrigation, and should be wide enough to allow space for elevation of the root to be removed. The remaining portion of tooth should be relieved of eccentric occlusal contact if it appears very mobile after surgery.

Tunnel Preparation

An alternative to root resection, in the case of lower molars with widely separated roots, may be tunnel preparation. This is a

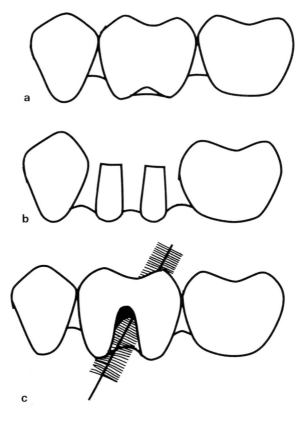

Fig. 11.5   (a) *Lower first molar has a furcation lesion Grade II/III.*
(b) *Endodontic treatment followed by periodontal surgery with
separation of mesial and distal roots has been carried out.*
(c) *Function is restored by means of a 'double crown', which admits
an interdental brush.*

surgical procedure involving removal of inter-radicular tissue to
accommodate an oral hygiene aid. However, only with long
roots can a tunnel be produced which will be large enough to
admit an interdental brush since, after healing, the inter-
radicular gingiva will tend to occupy about 4 mm of vertical
space coronal to the remaining bone. An interdental brush will
require a further 2–3 mm. This difficulty may be overcome by
separating the roots and providing a higher roof for the furcation
by means of a 'double crown' (Fig. 11.5). A significant

disadvantage of tunnel preparation appears to be a high caries risk.

Palliative Maintenance/Extraction

Often teeth with Grade II or Grade III involvement will require either extraction or palliative treatment by maintaining oral hygiene as far as possible, while recognising that gradual deterioration is likely. Such teeth may be usefully maintained for many years but are unpredictable in this respect. Seldom can their use as bridge abutments be justified, but they may be employed as partial-denture abutments and may allow a free-end saddle design to be avoided. If possible, some provision should be made in the denture design for addition of such a tooth should extraction become inevitable.

PROGNOSIS

The preservation of connective tissue attachment around the roots of multirooted teeth depends on elimination of plaque, calculus and contaminated cementum and subsequent establishment of a gingival contour which can be maintained plaque-free (Hamp *et al.*, 1975). In the case of extensive lesions, this may be possible only if roots are resected to eliminate inaccessible areas of plaque accumulation and so prognosis may also depend on satisfactory endodontic treatment. The periodontal prognosis will be best if root resection is carried out early, that is, as soon as plaque and/or calculus in furcation areas cannot be removed by scalers or curettes (Waerhaug, 1980). However, as already stated, limited resources preclude the wide application of such techniques and, therefore, many teeth are either extracted or maintained palliatively. It should be noted, in this regard, that Ross and Thomson (1978, 1980) and Knowles *et al.* (1980) have reported satisfactory maintenance of furcation-involved teeth without resorting to root resection.

Teeth with uncertain prognosis can be retained provided:

a) the uncertainty is acknowledged;
b) the patient is symptom-free—there is no discomfort or gross discharge;
c) there are no signs of rapid bone loss such as increasing mobility.

PREVENTION

Much of the prevention of furcation involvement applies equally to all marginal periodontal disease. The following list will serve to emphasise the main principles.

a) Interdental plaque control measures should be introduced early.
b) Diagnosis of marginal disease should be made early.
c) Posterior teeth should be scaled very thoroughly.
d) Matrix bands should be adequately wedged.
e) As far as possible, restoration margins should be supragingival. Subgingival extension 'for prevention of caries' will merely promote periodontal disease.
f) Approximal contact areas should be maintained when restoring a proximal surface.

REFERENCES

Hamp S.-E., Nyman S., Lindhe J. (1975). Periodontal treatment of multi-rooted teeth. *Journal of Clinical Periodontology*; **2**: 126–35.

Knowles J., Burgett F., Morrison E., Nissle R., Ramfjord S. (1980). Comparison of results following three modalities of periodontal therapy related to tooth type. *Journal of Clinical Periodontology*; **7**: 32–47.

Nyman S., Lindhe J. (1976). Considerations in the treatment of patients with multiple teeth with furcation involvements. *Journal of Clinical Periodontology*; **3**: 4–13.

Ross I., Thomson R. (1978). A long-term study of root retention in the treatment of maxillary molars with furcation involvement. *Journal of Periodontology*; **49**: 238–44.

Ross I., Thomson R. (1980). Furcation involvement in maxillary and mandibular molars. *Journal of Periodontology*; **51**: 450–4.

Waerhaug J. (1980). The furcation problem. Etiology, pathogenesis, diagnosis, therapy and prognosis. *Journal of Clinical Periodontology*; **7**: 73–95.

FURTHER READING

Newell D. (1981). Current status of the management of teeth with furcation invasions. *Journal of Periodontology*; **52**: 559–68.

Nordland P., Garret S., Kiger R., Vanooteghem R., Hutchens L. H., Egelberg J. (1987). The effect of plaque control and root debridement in molar teeth. *Journal of Clinical Periodontology*; **14**: 231–6.

Chapter 12

Periodontal–Pulpal Relationships

The purpose of this chapter is to review the aetiology and management of lesions which may result from communication and spread of inflammation between pulp and periodontium. Potential pathways for initiation or spread of inflammation are:

a) dentinal tubules;
b) lateral and accessory root canals;
c) the apical foramen;
d) cracks and fracture lines;
e) iatrogenic perforations.

CLASSIFICATION OF COMBINED LESIONS

A simple classification forms a basis for a rational approach to diagnosis and treatment planning for combined periodontal–pulpal lesions.

1. Periodontal disease with secondary pulp involvement.
2. Pulp disease with secondary periodontal involvement.
3. 'True' combined lesions where coincidental lesions of periodontal and pulpal origin have enlarged and merged.

AETIOLOGY

The dental pulp has a limited capacity to respond to noxious stimuli and loss of vitality may be caused by caries, abrasion, restorative procedures and materials, thermal changes, trauma and the toxic effects of bacterial plaque. In some cases, pulp changes may reflect the cumulative effect of several stimuli.

1. Periodontal disease leading to secondary pulp involvement (Fig. 12.1). Gingival recession may expose dentine tubules to the oral environment and hence the pulp to the aforementioned irritants. Whether the resulting pulp changes are reversible or lead to progressive pulp necrosis will depend on the initial status of the pulp, the severity of the stimulus and any concurrent stimuli.

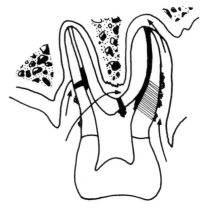

Fig. 12.1 *Periodontal disease with secondary pulp involvement. Pulp may be affected via apical, lateral or accessory (furcation) canals or via dentine tubules.*

Within periodontal pockets, plaque bacteria and their toxins may come in contact with dentinal tubules. This may occur because of the permeability of cementum or as a result of cementum removal during treatment exposing the underlying dentine. Similarly, both periodontal lesions and therapy may involve lateral canals or fracture lines associated with hitherto vital pulp tissue.

Periodontal occlusal trauma, at least in theory, may cause pulp ischaemia, especially in teeth with greatly reduced periodontal support.

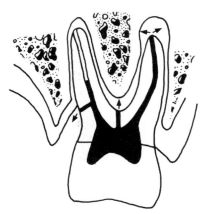

Fig. 12.2 *Pulp disease with secondary periodontal involvement via apical, lateral and accessory (furcation) canals.*

2. Pulp disease leading to secondary periodontal involvement (Fig. 12.2). Egress of bacteria, toxins and products of pulp necrosis from apical foramina frequently leads to an acute or chronic periapical area of destruction of periodontal membrane and adjacent bone. The same process may occur at lateral or accessory canals, and adjacent to fracture lines and perforations such as may occur during endodontic treatment or post preparation. The inflammatory process may lead to a discharge through the marginal periodontium, inviting the misdiagnosis of a pocket of periodontal origin.

3. 'True' combined lesions (Fig. 12.3). In these cases there is no clear indication from history or examintion of an aetiological link between the lesions of marginal periodontium and endodontic origin. A true combined lesion is, therefore, best regarded as two separate lesions which have enlarged and merged.

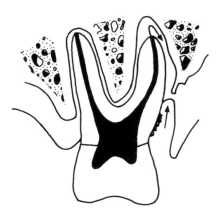

Fig. 12.3   *True combined lesion. Lesions of apical and marginal origin communicate at the base of a deep periodontal pocket.*

DIAGNOSIS

A careful history of onset and development of signs and symptoms should be taken and followed by clinical examination, radiographs and vitality tests. It may not be possible, however, to obtain a clear history for chronic symptomless periodontal–pulpal lesions. Diagnosis is generally easier during or just after an acute episode.

Clinical Examination

One should be alerted to the possibility of periodontal–pulpal communication by discoloured clinical crowns, sinuses, gross gingival exudate and probing levels which seem to be uncharacteristic of the general condition of the mouth. It should be apparent that, because of the cumulative effect of various noxious stimuli on the pulp, heavily restored teeth with significant attachment loss due to periodontal disease are more likely to be non-vital and exhibit combined lesions.

When a lesion of endodontic origin spreads to involve a previously healthy marginal periodontium, probing may reveal a very narrow defect of depth atypical of the general level of periodontal destruction. Moreover, such root surfaces are likely to be relatively free of subgingival deposits unless the lesion is of long standing.

Pockets due to marginal periodontal disease usually possess a wide gingival orifice and deposits of calculus may be detected on the root surface. In addition, in established cases the probing depths tend to be greatest interdentally, with relative health buccally and lingually. Teeth are very rarely affected in isolation.

One must be wary to distinguish the drainage of infection through the cortical plate apically, then subperiosteally to the gingival margin, without destruction of marginal periodontium. This distinction should be possible by careful probing.

Vitality Testing

The response of the pulp to vitality testing depends on an intact nerve supply, whereas vitality may in fact be maintained by blood supply alone. Testing may be carried out electrically, thermally and by tactile stimulus with probe or bur. None of these tests is infallible and both false positive and false negative responses may be found. This is particularly likely in heavily restored teeth and in multirooted teeth.

Radiographic Examination

This has been discussed in Chapter 5. It will suffice to remind the reader that a careful check should be made for widening of periodontal membrane space or loss of lamina dura, in addition to larger apical or lateral areas of rarefaction. Lesions may be masked by superimposition and their size is likely to be underestimated. Lateral and accessory canals and fracture lines may be invisible. Furcation radiolucency may be endodontic in origin.

Correlation of Diagnostic Findings

A careful analysis of all available data will usually clarify the diagnosis. However, it may be impossible to establish the nature of a combined lesion particularly when of long duration. The patient should be advised of this but, for treatment planning purposes, where doubt exists, the lesion should be considered endodontic in origin.

HEALING POTENTIAL

As stated in Chapter 7, the healing of endodontic lesions without marginal involvement is predictable if adequate endodontic treatment is carried out, and can be expected to result in regeneration of bone and periodontal membrane. This is because epithelium is normally excluded from the area. Regeneration of marginal periodontium, however, appears to be possible only to a very limited extent owing to the pathological and therapeutic alteration of tooth surface and the rapid migration of epithelium along the root. The healing of combined lesions is therefore less predictable, as the proportion of periodontal destruction due to each process may be unclear and, in any case, chronic lesions of endodontic origin are likely to become plaque-infected and cementum pathologically altered. Whatever potential for regeneration may exist should be fully exploited, and so endodontic treatment should precede periodontal treatment. In any case, periodontal treatment is destined to fail while infection of endodontic origin persists.

TREATMENT

1. Periodontal disease with secondary pulp involvement. Periodontal disease is almost invariably chronic, although acute disease may be superimposed. Secondary pulp involvement may range from a mild reversible pulpitis to progressive necrosis.

The treatment of periodontal disease is described in other chapters. Furthermore, when dentine sensitivity occurs as a result of gingival recession, it should be treated as soon as possible by applications of fluoride varnish or other desensitising agents. Failure to recognise this problem may lead to inhibition of tooth cleaning and plaque accumulation. This, in turn, may cause pulpal hyperaemia or early pulpitis and, indeed, increased hypersensitivity.

If periodontal disease leads to irreversible pulpitis or pulp necrosis, endodontic treatment should be carried out before periodontal treatment.

2. Pulp disease with secondary periodontal involvement. In these cases, the pulp disease will have progressed at least to partial necrosis and will necessitate endodontic treatment. Whether subsequent conventional periodontal treatment is required will depend on the duration of communication with the gingival margin or base of any existing pocket. Thus, when duration of communication is short (because of early diagnosis), plaque contamination of the root surface is less likely to have occurred and regeneration can be expected.

On the other hand, communication between endodontic and marginal lesions of long duration is more likely to result in accumulation of plaque and calculus with alteration of cementum. These lesions are more likely to require extensive débridement, possibly with surgical access. Nevertheless, such cases should invariably first have endodontic treatment, to exploit fully the potential for the marginal tissues to heal.

3. 'True' combined lesions. Endodontic treatment should be carried out first, following the same principles as in 1 and 2 above.

FURCATION LESIONS

A high incidence of accessory pulp canals has been reported in the furcations of multirooted teeth. When a furcation lesion is diagnosed, vitality testing should be employed and non-vital teeth treated endodontically, with a special search made of the floor of the pulp chamber for accessory canals. Furcation lesions of endodontic origin may be expected to heal if root canal therapy is carried out at an early stage.

IATROGENIC LESIONS

These are usually endodontic in origin with secondary periodontal involvement such as may occur with overfilling of root canals or perforation with root canal instruments or burs, usually during post-crown preparation. It is important that any such problems be recognised early and the patient advised. Signs and symptoms should be monitored carefully before further treatment is undertaken.

The prognosis for perforated roots is closely related to size and position. Small perforations in the apical third may be amenable to retrograde filling or apicectomy. In the mid-third, perforations on the labial aspect will be accessible and should be repaired early with amalgam; prognosis is good if marginal communication is avoided. In the coronal third, marginal communication is likely to persist, i.e. a pocket may have to be accepted. Palatal and proximal surface perforations in the coronal two-thirds are likely to be inaccessible or necessitate removal of too much supporting bone to gain access. Such teeth should be kept under review or extracted.

FURTHER READING

Gold S. I., Moskow B. S. (1987). Periodontal repair of periapical lesions: the borderland between pulpal and periodontal disease. *Journal of Clinical Periodontology*; **14**: 251–6.

Harrington G. W. (1979). The perio-endo question: differential diagnosis. *Dental Clinics of North America*; **23**: 673–90.

Hiatt W. H. (1977). Pulpal periodontal disease. *Journal of Periodontology*; **48**: 598–609.

Stallard R. E. (1972). Periodontic-endodontic relationships. *Oral Surgery*; **34**: 314–25.

Stock C. J. R. (1985). Calcium hydroxide: root resorption and perio-endo lesions. *British Dental Journal*; **158**: 325–34.

Tidmarsh B. G. (1979). Accidental perforation of the roots of teeth. *Journal of Oral Rehabilitation*; **6**: 235–40.

Zamet J. S. (1976). Periodontal disease and the dental pulp. In *Endodontics in Clinical Practice*. (Harty F. J., ed.) pp. 226–40. Bristol: John Wright.

Chapter 13

Mucogingival Problems

Attached gingiva is well adapted to withstand frictional stresses from the passage of food and the use of the toothbrush, and to dissipate pull from the lip and cheek musculature. Alveolar mucosa is structured to facilitate jaw movement. This chapter evaluates the significance of an 'adequate' width of attached gingiva in the maintenance of periodontal health.

DETERMINANTS OF WIDTH OF ATTACHED GINGIVA

The width of attached gingiva in the developing dentition is determined by hereditary factors, including growth of the alveolar process, position of teeth within the arch and location of fraenal insertion. There is great variation in width of attached gingiva between and within individuals. Occasionally there is no attached gingiva at all, usually because of high fraenal insertion (*see* Fig. 13.3). Attached gingiva, therefore, may be inherently deficient or may be reduced in width by gingival recession (*see* Fig. 13.10).

AETIOLOGY OF RECESSION

Position of Tooth in the Arch

Teeth which are prominent buccally or lingually in relation to the rest of the arch possess an inherent tendency for gingival recession. Such roots may have a relative lack of bony covering and there may be a long suprabony soft-tissue attachment (Fig. 13.1). Likewise, a thin interradicular septum between roots in close proximity may be subject to breakdown.

Inflammation

Gingival recession commonly accompanies plaque-induced chronic periodontal disease, possibly due to breakdown of

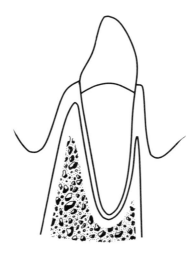

Fig. 13.1 *Lower canine in a prominent position, showing a relative lack of buccal supporting bone and a long soft-tissue attachment.*

connective tissue and subsidence of the epithelial surface—a process described more fully later in this chapter. This is probably the commonest explanation for interdental gingival recession.

Trauma

A single traumatic incident may inflict severe damage to the gingiva, leading to recession. This is relatively uncommon, however, compared to the incidence of chronic minor trauma and associated recession.

Trauma from oral hygiene devices. There is good circumstantial evidence that the toothbrush is a frequent cause of recession affecting buccal and lingual surfaces. Presumably, the force applied, the speed and frequency of brushing, the texture of the brush and abrasion from toothpaste are important factors. Trauma caused solely by the toothbrush is usually associated with good buccal and lingual plaque control, gingival health and smooth, highly-polished tooth surfaces. Cervical abrasion cavities may be present.

Interdental toothbrushes or woodpoints, used injudiciously, may cause interdental recession.

Other forms of self-inflicted trauma. Children or adolescents may exhibit gingival ulceration and recession due to repeated injury from the habitual use of fingernails, pencils, etc.

Impaired food shedding. The cervical bulge of a tooth will normally deflect food away from the gingival margin. If, however, the tooth is malaligned the protective effect of the cervical bulge will be lost on one surface. Likewise, under-contoured restorations may allow food impingement against the gingival margin.

Occlusal trauma.

a) Tooth–soft-tissue contacts. Excessive incisor overlap may allow the upper incisors to 'strip' the lower labial gingiva or the lower incisors to 'strip' the upper palatal gingiva. Food will impinge against the gingival margin during mastication. Furthermore, clenching or grinding habits may permit attrition and over-eruption, perpetuating the soft-tissue trauma.

b) Tooth–tooth contacts. The traditional view that gingival recession is a direct result of occlusal trauma has not been substantiated. On the other hand, tooth movement may occur as an adaptive response to occlusal trauma. Depending on the nature of the forces, this may result in migration or mobility and, perhaps, in bony dehiscence, a factor which may predispose to subsequent gingival recession.

Removable prostheses. Without adequate tooth support removable prostheses may sink into the gingival tissue, causing recession. Alternatively, they may cause tooth movement. Much of the recession may also be attributable to the inflammatory changes caused by increased plaque accumulation beneath the denture.

Surgical pocket therapy. Gingival recession is an inevitable consequence of all forms of surgical pocket therapy, but especially the gingivectomy and apically repositioned flap procedures.

PATHOGENESIS OF RECESSION

Baker and Seymour (1976) have presented a hypothesis on the development of gingival recession, based on histological studies

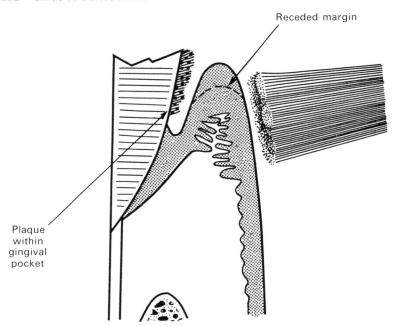

Receded margin

Plaque
within
gingival
pocket

Fig. 13.2   *Hypothetical explanation of gingival recession. Two possible inflammatory stimuli, either plaque or toothbrushing, may lead to the lateral extension of rete pegs and the formation of an interconnecting cord of epithelium. This may be followed by subsidence of the epithelial surface.*

of experimental recession in the rat. Briefly, it is explained as follows.

The connective tissues underlying oral epithelium may become inflamed owing to physical irritation (e.g. toothbrushing). The connective tissue underlying pocket epithelium may be the seat of an inflammatory process because of plaque on the tooth surface. Inflammatory processes lead to connective tissue destruction. Epithelial cells tend to proliferate into the connective tissue until, as a result of rete peg elongation, an interconnecting cord of epithelium is formed between the oral and pocket epithelia (Fig. 13.2). This is followed by subsidence of the epithelial surface which is manifest clinically as recession. Recession may, therefore, be due entirely to bacterial plaque or physical trauma or it may be a combination of these two factors. Furthermore, gingiva which is thin buccolingually will be at greater risk of recession.

Although the entire width of attached gingiva may be destroyed, a narrow zone of keratinised tissue, i.e. free gingiva will tend to be retained (Wennström and Lindhe, 1983), owing to the keratinising influence of the periodontal membrane on overlying epithelium (*see below*).

CLINICAL SIGNIFICANCE OF MINIMAL WIDTH OF ATTACHED GINGIVA

It has recently been shown from numerous experimental studies that: with good plaque control, gingivitis will not occur, irrespective of the presence or absence of attached gingiva; the inflammatory lesion in the gingiva which follows plaque accumulation is not enhanced in cases where the zone of attached gingiva is very narrow or missing altogether; gingival recession is *not* more likely to occur in areas with minimal width of gingiva than in areas of considerable width. This would indicate that there is no such thing as a minimum required width of attached gingiva, and that attached gingiva is *not* required to support the junctional epithelium, allowing it to maintain a seal against the tooth surface during function, as was once thought.

The presence, therefore, of a deficient band of attached gingiva should not give cause for concern *unless* the peculiar tissue morphology prohibits satisfactory plaque control, leading to

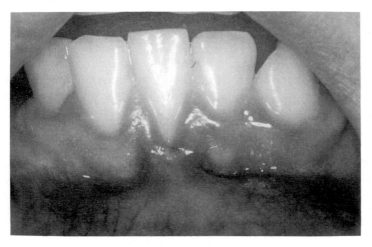

Fig. 13.3 *A high fraenal attachment reduces access for toothbrushing.*

chronic periodontal disease. Particular difficulty with oral hygiene may be experienced when a fraenum is attached at the gingival margin (Fig. 13.3). Teeth tend to be affected singly. The patient may modify his toothbrushing technique to avoid traumatising the non-keratinised alveolar mucosa and fail to achieve complete plaque removal.

If gingival recession has occurred, it is likely to cease when thicker mucosa is reached. If plaque accumulation persists, however, periodontal breakdown may continue with the development of pockets.

TREATMENT OF MUCOGINGIVAL PROBLEMS

Where gingivitis or periodontitis occurs in areas of minimal gingival width, the first line of treatment involves scaling and root planing, if necessary, and instruction in an efficient but atraumatic brushing technique. The single-tufted toothbrush is often helpful. In the majority of cases, no further treatment is necessary.

Where an inflammatory lesion occurs in association with gingival recession, a small amount of coronal gingival regrowth may occur with the establishment of periodontal health. To prevent further recession, all aetiological factors should be eliminated as far as possible. This means that, in addition to teaching an effective, atraumatic cleaning technique, other sources of trauma should be eliminated; displaced, migrated or hypermobile teeth may require stabilisation within the arch.

When, in spite of careful instruction, patients remain unable to perform adequate oral hygiene owing to abnormal mucogingival relationships, surgical intervention should be considered. There are essentially three treatment options.

a)   Gingival extension surgery to create a deepened vestibule and a functional width of attached gingiva, apical to the original mucogingival junction. 'Functional', in this context, refers to the need for a band of gingiva which will allow toothbrushing without discomfort. Gingival extension is, nowadays, usually achieved by the free gingival graft technique (Fig. 13.4). This method is applicable to teeth affected by recession as well as those with an inherent lack of attached gingiva.

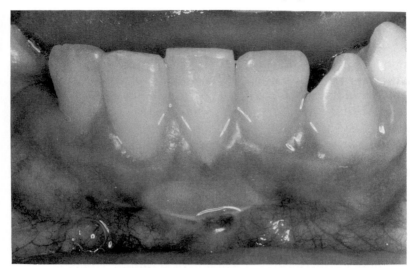

Fig. 13.4 *Free gingival graft employed in situation illustrated by Fig. 13.3. Note, however, that patient's toothbrushing habits have not altered and gingivitis is still present.*

b) Laterally transposed flap to restore a covering of gingiva to the exposed root surface in cases of gingival recession.

c) A combination of (a) and (b), where a free gingival graft is first carried out, followed, at a later appointment, by a coronally sliding flap procedure which covers the exposed root in cases of gingival recession.

These modes of therapy may be described as *mucogingival surgery*, i.e. their prime aim is to alter mucogingival relationships rather than treat a gingival or periodontal pocket.

Gingival Extension

A wide variety of techniques has been described for vestibular deepening and/or gingival extension, namely: vestibuloplasty; sulcus deepening; periosteal separation; fraenectomy etc. Essentially, these involved an incision along the mucogingival junction followed by a sharp dissection, severing muscle and connective tissue attachments from the periosteum, until the desired depth of sulcus was achieved. Denudation of alveolar bone, instead of periosteal retention, was also attempted. These techniques, although simple to perform, gave rise to significant postoperative pain and swelling. Healing was prolonged and scarring was common. Substantial resorption of alveolar bone occurred with denudation techniques. The 'periosteal separation' technique emerged as one of the better options. Even so, only a narrow band of new gingiva could be created, with poor predictability. These techniques are now mainly of historical interest and have been superseded by the free gingival graft technique. A comparative study is reported by Jenkins and Stephen (1979).

Biological rationale of the free gingival graft. The potential for epithelium to keratinise depends, not on functional demands, but mainly on the inherited characteristics of the underlying connective tissue (for review, see Heaney, 1974). Non-keratinised epithelium will not necessarily keratinise when exposed to friction. Hence the failure of alveolar mucosa to keratinise as gingival recession approaches the mucogingival junction. Furthermore, a transplant of keratinised mucosa, when

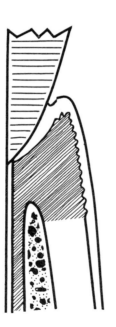 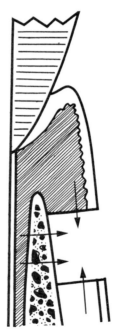

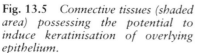

Fig. 13.5 *Connective tissues (shaded area) possessing the potential to induce keratinisation of overlying epithelium.*

Fig. 13.6 *The origin of granulation tissue in the repair of an alveolar mucosal wound.*

located within the alveolar mucosa, i.e. an environment where keratinisation is normally absent, will retain its keratinising ability owing to the influence of the transplanted connective tissue. This is the rationale behind the free gingival graft procedure. The description of the principles of successful grafting by Sullivan and Atkins (1968*a*) is recommended.

The inability of certain connective tissues to induce keratinisation of overlying epithelium, also explains the failure of the earlier vestibuloplasty techniques to produce a predictable band of keratinised tissue, apical to the mucogingival junction. Figure 13.5 illustrates those connective tissues in the environment of the tooth which possess the potential to induce keratinisation of overlying epithelium. Figure 13.6 shows the various sources of granulation tissue which form the healing wound. Ironically, it can be seen that the maximum amount of keratinised tissue will develop when postoperative resorption of supporting bone occurs, allowing the periodontal membrane connective tissues to reach the wound surface to contribute to the formation of new keratinised gingiva. This concept of wound healing is based on the work of Karring *et al.* (1975).

Free gingival graft—outline of the technique.

a) An incision is made at the mucogingival line (Fig. 13.7).
b) A mucosal flap is produced, to an apical extension of about 6–8 mm. A thin layer of periosteum should be retained over the bone (Fig. 13.8).

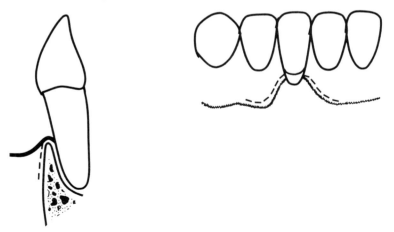

Fig. 13.7 *Free gingival graft procedure: the initial incision.*

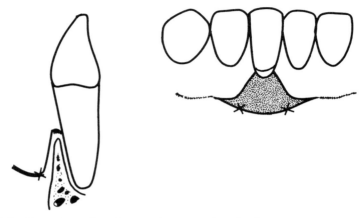

Fig. 13.8 *Free gingival graft procedure: suturing the flap.*

c) The flap margin should be sutured to its base (Fig. 13.8).
d) Scaling and root planing is carried out.
e) The periosteal bed, which will receive the graft, will usually be triangular in outline. A piece of tin foil is cut to size to occupy a slightly smaller area than the underlying periosteum. The tin foil becomes a template for the graft.
f) The donor site is usually in the second premolar/first molar region of the palate, just behind the rugae, and as close to the palatal gingival margins of these teeth as is practicable. An incision is made round the tin foil template to a depth of about 1·25–1·5 mm, i.e. extending to the full thickness of the mucosa but without including a significant amount of submucosa. Such a graft, consisting of epithelium plus the full amount of lamina propria, would be termed a full-thickness graft. The tin foil template is removed and the graft tissue dissected out. Any adherent fatty or glandular tissue should be scraped from the graft. An alternative, faster technique for removing the graft is by excision with a Pacquette knife, although the tissue so obtained requires trimming to fit the recipient site.
g) The graft is transferred to the recipient site and held in place with as few sutures as possible to avoid unnecessary trauma (Fig. 13.9).
h) Pressure over the graft for two to three minutes will expel

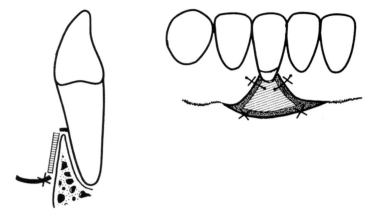

Fig. 13.9 *Free gingival graft procedure: suturing the graft.*

blood from the wound and stabilise the graft prior to application of a Coe-pak® dressing.

i) The donor site is protected by an acrylic plate, manufactured from a preoperative impression. This is the surest way to reduce postoperative pain and prevent haemorrhage. The plate may be lined in the wound area with Coe-pak® or tissue conditioner.

j) Dressing and sutures are removed after one week and the patient advised to avoid brushing the area of the graft for two to four weeks. Chlorhexidine mouthwash is prescribed during this time. Although graft epithelium usually desquamates, it is recolonised by epithelium from adjacent tissues, with keratinisation occurring in four weeks.

Free gingival graft—wound healing. Survival of the graft in the first two postoperative days is solely dependent on a plasmatic circulation, i.e. diffusion of nutrients from the host bed. Thereafter, a capillary network extends into the graft. As a rule, free graft tissue placed over a root surface will undergo necrosis through lack of nutrient diffusion, unless the area of recession is narrow and a significant amount of graft tissue lies on either side of the 'bridge' to provide a collateral source of diffused nutrient. The free gingival graft, therefore, has a limited potential to cover the exposed root surface. The prospects of covering a denuded root surface by 'bridging' with a free graft are discussed by Sullivan and Atkins (1968b).

The Laterally Transposed Flap

This is a pedicle graft by which coverage of a denuded root can be predictably achieved in suitably selected cases. The graft is maintained by its own blood supply while adhesion to the root surface occurs. This involves epithelial down-growth on the inner surface of the flap and the formation of a long junctional epithelium which forms an epithelial attachment.

There are two major drawbacks to this method of providing a functional width of gingiva. At the *donor* site, healing may be complicated by recession; at the *recipient* site, further recession is likely unless the cause of the original recession is identified and eliminated, and, since recession tends to occur over prominent root surfaces, orthodontic treatment will be necessary in many cases to reposition the tooth prior to mucogingival surgery.

These considerations severely limit the applicability of this procedure, and, in most instances, the free gingival graft procedure is to be preferred as a means of providing a functional width of gingiva, even although little root coverage is achieved.

Free Gingival Graft with Coronally Repositioned Flap

This is a two-stage procedure with the ultimate aim of covering an exposed root surface. It will not be described at length here. Initially, a free gingival graft is placed to extend the gingiva apically. Then, about two months later, a flap is raised and advanced coronally over the exposed root.

This procedure avoids one of the drawbacks of the laterally transposed flap—the risk of recession at the donor site. On the other hand, an additional surgical insult is necessary. The procedure was developed originally to allow coverage of multiple adjacent denuded roots. However, mucogingival surgery for more than one tooth unit is rarely required, and this two-stage procedure would appear to have very little application.

CONCLUSION

Mucogingival surgery has generated a substantial literature which seems to overstate the frequency and importance of mucogingival problems. The following should be remembered.

a)   There is no basis for the belief that extending the width of a

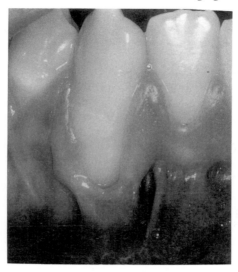

Fig. 13.10 *Clinically healthy gingiva in spite of unfavourable mucogingival relationships in 3̄ region. This patient has learned to overcome the difficulty of cleaning the cervical portion of this tooth.*

narrow band of gingiva will prevent further recession. Neither can one confidently assume that the coverage of a denuded root surface will not be followed by recurrent recession.

b) When attached gingiva is deficient, plaque control in the cervical tooth region may become difficult owing to the proximity of alveolar mucosa. Gingivitis may supervene. However, scaling and oral hygiene instruction is often rewarded by the establishment of gingival health (Fig. 13.10).

c) Mucogingival surgery should be reserved for cases where good plaque control and gingival health cannot be secured because of an unfavourable mucogingival environment. The technique of choice will usually be the free gingival graft.

REFERENCES

Baker D. L., Seymour G. J. (1976). The possible pathogenesis of gingival recession. A histological study of induced recession in the rat. *Journal of Clinical Periodontology*; 3: 208–19.

Heaney T. G. (1974). A reappraisal of environment, function and gingival specificity. *Journal of Periodontology*; **45**: 695–700.

Jenkins W. M . M., Stephen K. W. (1979). A clinical comparison of two gingival extension procedures. *Journal of Dentistry*; 7: 91–7.

Karring T., Cumming B. R., Oliver R. C., Loe H. (1975). The origin of granulation tissue and its impact on post-operative results of mucogingival surgery. *Journal of Periodontology*; **46**: 577–85.

Sullivan H. C., Atkins J. H. (1968*a*). Free autogenous gingival grafts I. Principles of successful grafting. *Periodontics*; **6**: 121–9.

Sullivan H. C., Atkins J. H. (1968*b*). Free autogenous gingival grafts III. Utilization of grafts in the treatment of gingival recession. *Periodontics*; **6**: 152–60.

Wennström J., Lindhe J. (1983). Role of attached gingiva for maintenance of periodontal health. *Journal of Clinical Periodontology*; **10**: 206–21.

FURTHER READING

Addy M., Dummer P. M. H., Hunter M. L., Kingdon A., Shaw W. C. (1987). A study of the association of fraenal attachment, lip coverage, and vestibular depth with plaque and gingivitis. *Journal of Periodontology*; **58**: 752–7.

Eaton K. A., Kieser J. B. (1986). A conservative approach to the management of gingival recession and other gingival 'inadequacy'. *Restorative Dentistry*; **2**: 29–35.

Lange D. E. (1985). Indications and procedures for mucogingival surgery. In *Orthodontics and Periodontics*. (Hosl E., Zachrisson B. U., Baldauf A., eds.) pp. 79–103. Chicago: Quintessence.

Chapter 14

Juvenile Periodontitis

DEFINITION

Juvenile periodontitis, formerly known as periodontosis, is a rapidly destructive disease of the periodontal tissues with its onset in puberty. It affects otherwise healthy individuals or, at any rate, individuals in whom systemic disease is purely coincidental. Similar destructive changes may occur in juveniles affected by a variety of systemic diseases. By definition, however, the periodontal diagnosis in these cases is not juvenile periodontitis.

PREVALENCE

The disease occurs in approximtely 1 in 1000 adolescents. There seems to be a racial predisposition, individuals of African or Asian origin being more frequently affected. Early reports of a predilection for girls are at variance with more recent evidence suggesting an equal incidence in both sexes.

CLINICAL FEATURES

Unlike adult chronic periodontitis, the prevalence and severity of which is broadly related to standards of oral hygiene, juvenile periodontitis may affect relatively clean as well as dirty mouths. When oral hygiene is poor, connective tissue attachment loss will be accompanied by frank gingivitis. On the other hand, in relatively clean mouths, gingivitis may be virtually absent, masking the presence of underlying destructive lesions. The condition is often brought to the patient's attention by the development of tooth mobility or migration or the occurrence of a periodontal abscess, all signs of advanced destruction.

Initially, first permanent molars and permanent incisors are affected (Fig. 14.1) although, ultimately, the appearance may be that of generalised advanced attachment loss. As the disease

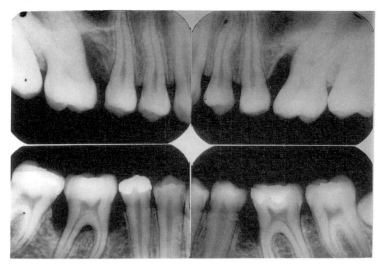

Fig. 14.1 *Juvenile periodontitis principally affecting the first molars in a 16-year-old. The lower incisors were affected to a minor degree.*

progresses it usually exhibits a roughly symmetrical pattern of tooth involvement. The incisor/molar pattern of involvement is probably a reflection of their earlier eruption times and the fact that they have been exposed longer to the oral environment. 'Localised juvenile periodontitis' is an expression sometimes used to describe cases where only incisors and first permanent molars are affected.

AETIOLOGY

The disease appears to be inherited. Although the primary hereditary defect is unknown, this seems to be manifest as a gross imbalance of host–parasite equilibrium so that, following a short period of exposure to small amounts of plaque, a destructive lesion develops.

MICROBIOLOGY

Subgingival plaque is present as a thin Gram-negative layer, loosely attached to the tooth surface. It differs markedly from adult chronic periodontitis where a comparatively thick subgingival flora is present. The subgingival flora of juvenile periodontitis has a variable composition and may include any of the putative pathogens described in Table 20.1. However, *Actinobacillus actinomycetemcomitans*, a capnophilic non-motile rod, is isolated more frequently and often in greater proportions than it is from adult periodontitis lesions. This organism possesses numerous virulence factors. A potent leukotoxin, for example, is produced by many strains of *A. actinomycetemcomitans* causing neutrophil and monocyte lysis. Furthermore, there is some evidence, not fully substantiated, that *A. actinomycetemcomitans* may be capable of invading pocket soft tissues. This could have implications for treatment (*see below*).

Subgingival calculus is virtually absent in juvenile periodontitis.

HOST DEFENCE MECHANISMS

Juvenile periodontitis patients may exhibit an impaired lymphocyte blastogenic response in the presence of host Gram-negative micro-organisms. Furthermore, there is considerable evidence of inherited chemotactic defects in circulating neutrophils of individuals suffering from juvenile periodontitis. Monocyte chemotaxis may also be affected. Why these individuals fail to show impaired general health is not clear, but it has been suggested that subgingival plaque bacteria, in contrast to many other bacteria, are only mildly chemotactic and unable to attract defective neutrophils. The same neutrophils might be able to respond to the greater chemotactic stimuli of other pathogenic organisms.

HISTOPATHOLOGY

The histological picture is dominated by dense accumulation of plasma cells and blast cells in the infiltrated connective tissue. In the case of adult chronic periodontitis, a smaller proportion of inflammatory cells and a larger proportion of extracellular tissue is observed in the infiltrated area.

POSTJUVENILE PERIODONTITIS

The expression 'juvenile periodontitis' is usually reserved for cases which are identified by the age of 21 years (i.e. juveniles). Nevertheless, young adults over 21 years may also present a clinical picture of severe periodontal breakdown which is inconsistent with their standard of plaque control. This condition has been termed 'postjuvenile periodontitis' or, more recently, 'rapidly progressive periodontitis'. Unlike juvenile periodontitis, severe periodontitis in young adults lacks well-defined characteristics. Some of these patients may have had the disease during adolescence without it being diagnosed as juvenile periodontitis at that time. In others it appears to commence during early adult life. In some young adults, the disease is confined to first molars and incisors, but usually most, if not all, of the dentition is affected. Microbiological findings are variable and immunological abnormalities are not consistently found.

TREATMENT OF JUVENILE PERIODONTITIS

Treatment proceeds as for adult chronic periodontitis. However, even greater emphasis should be placed on the need for good supragingival plaque control by the patient and scrupulous attention to the subgingival environment by the clinician. Without thorough subgingival plaque control, which may require surgical access, the prognosis is poor. On the other hand, surgical intervention, where necessary, should be rewarded by rapid healing and more bone regeneration within angular bone defects than might be observed in the treatment of adult chronic periodontitis.

A number of studies have been carried out suggesting that a two to three week course of systemic tetracycline gives better results than instrumentation alone, whether non-surgical or surgical. The use of an antibiotic in these cases is based on the belief that *A. actinomycetemcomitans* is difficult to eradicate by instrumentation alone from periodontal tissues which it is thought to invade (*see* Chapter 20). Systemic tetracycline has been chosen because it is effective against *A. actinomycetemcomitans* and achieves high concentrations in gingival fluid. Several authors, on the other hand, have reported excellent results from conventional treatment without antibiotics in patients followed up for several years.

Although tetracycline has low toxicity, resistant bacterial strains develop readily. In view of this and in light of the conflicting evidence for its necessity in treatment of juvenile periodontitis, it would seem prudent to reserve tetracycline for patients for whom conventional treatment has been unsuccessful. If tetracycline therapy is provided, it should be accompanied by thorough mechanical débridement and must not be used in isolation.

The demonstration of specific defects of neutrophils or monocytes or of the immune system has little bearing on treatment, there being no real alternative to traditional forms of therapy at the present time.

OTHER CAUSES FOR ADVANCED PERIODONTAL DESTRUCTION IN CHILDREN

Although juvenile periodontitis is not associated with underlying systemic disease, it must be remembered that some cases of advanced chronic periodontitis are directly related to a number of uncommon or rare diseases which render the host more susceptible to bacterial plaque. These conditions include hypophosphatasia, Papillon–Lefèvre syndrome, agranulocytosis, cyclic neutropenia and leukaemia. Severe periodontal destruction in the primary dentition must certainly raise the suspicion of an underlying systemic disease. On the other hand, a few cases of advanced chronic periodontitis in otherwise healthy infants have been reported, although by definition these should not be described as juvenile periodontitis.

FURTHER READING

Burmeister J. A., Best A. M., Palcanis K. G., Caine F. A., Ranney R. R. (1984). Localized juvenile periodontitis and generalised severe periodontitis: clinical findings. *Journal of Clinical Periodontology*; **11**: 181–92.

Christersson L. A., Slots J., Rosling B. G., Genco R. J. (1985). Microbiological and clinical effects of surgical treatment of localized juvenile periodontitis. *Journal of Clinical Periodontology*; **12**: 465–76.

Davies R. M., Smith R. G., Porter S. R. (1985). Destructive forms of periodontal disease in adolescents and young adults. *British Dental Journal*; **158**: 429–36.

Gjermo P. (1986). Chemotherapy in juvenile periodontitis. *Journal of Clinical Periodontology*; **13**: 983–6.

Hormand J., Frandsen A. (1979). Juvenile periodontitis: localisation of bone loss in relation to age, sex and teeth. *Journal of Clinical Periodontology*; **6**: 407–16.

Liljenberg B., Lindhe J. (1980). Juvenile periodontitis: some micro-biological, histopathological and clinical characteristics. *Journal of Clinical Periodontology*; **7**: 48–61.

Lindhe J., Liljenberg B. (1984). Treatment of localized juvenile periodontitis. Results after 5 years. *Journal of Clinical Periodontology*; **11**: 399–410.

Saxby M. S. (1982). Juvenile periodontitis: an historical review. *Journal of Oral Rehabilitation*; **9**: 451–68.

Saxby M. S. (1987). Juvenile periodontitis: an epidemiological study in the west Midlands of the United Kingdom. *Journal of Clinical Periodontology*; **14**: 594–5.

Saxen L. (1980). Juvenile periodontitis: *Journal of Clinical Periodontology*; **7**: 1–19.

Waerhaug J. (1977). Plaque control in the treatment of juvenile periodontitis. *Journal of Clinical Periodontology*; **4**: 29–40.

Wennström A., Wennström J., Lindhe J. (1986). Healing following surgical and non-surgical treatment of juvenile periodontitis. A 5-year longitudinal study. *Journal of Clinical Periodontology*; **13**: 869–83.

Zambon J. J. (1985) *Actinobacillus actinomycetemcomitans* in human periodontal disease. *Journal of Clinical Periodontology*; **12**: 1–20.

Chapter 15

Occlusal Therapy

INTRODUCTION

Occlusal therapy in the periodontal context may be defined as any procedure which, by altering the direction, magnitude or distribution of occlusal forces, will reduce trauma or stabilise a tooth which is mobile or subject to migration. This may be achieved by reshaping occlusal surfaces (occlusal adjustment) or by increasing the tooth's resistance to applied force (splinting). The intention of this chapter is to put occlusal therapy in proper perspective in relation to periodontal disease and, therefore, only a brief description will be given of a few selected techniques of occlusal treatment. The reader is referred to Ramfjord and Ash (1983) for a detailed appraisal of occlusion. A series of papers on occlusion and restorative dentistry (Wise, 1986) is also recommended.

In the past, occlusal therapy has been a routine component of periodontal therapy, even though its rationale was uncertain. Yet occlusal therapy may be irreversible: most forms of occlusal adjustment and some forms of splinting involve destruction of tooth substance. Occlusal therapy, moreover, may focus patient attention on occlusion and away from plaque control. It is now recognised that this mode of treatment, so far as periodontal problems are concerned, should be reserved for a few well-defined situations.

INDICATIONS

The following is a list of the main indications for occlusal therapy:

a) progressive occlusal trauma
   i) surface injury (e.g. deep traumatic overbite and food impaction)
   ii) injury to the supporting structures
b) tooth hypermobility (if it interferes with patient comfort)
c) tooth migration

Of course, further indications for occlusal treatment exist in other areas of dentistry. For example, occlusal adjustment may be an important prelude to restorative treatment from simple restorations to complex fixed prosthodontics. In those situations, however, occlusal adjustment is intended primarily to facilitate the construction of satisfactory restorations and control the risk of technical failure, rather than directly to benefit the periodontium.

In every case (a–c) an occlusal aetiology must be demonstrable for occlusal therapy to be effective. Failure to observe this rule may result in unjustified mutilation of the occlusion. Tooth mobility, for example, is an inevitable consequence of marginal periodontitis, sooner or later, and it may persist even after successful treatment to arrest periodontal disease. A belief that any tooth mobility is unacceptable or necessarily a sign of poor prognosis may lead either to overtreatment by means of occlusal therapy or even to unnecessary tooth extraction. Most tooth mobility should be regarded as a sign of a reduced periodontium and appropriate steps should be taken to ensure control of inflammatory periodontal disease as a first priority. Only if mobility interferes with patient comfort or appears to be increasing in the absence of ongoing inflammatory periodontal disease, should occlusal therapy be considered, subject to the demonstration of a relevant occlusal abnormality.

Unwarranted occlusal therapy may also arise from the operator's desire to eliminate occlusal disharmony in spite of the absence of any pathological process. It should be borne in mind that occlusal abnormalities in the form of centric interferences are exceedingly common, as are clenching and grinding habits, which influence the magnitude and duration of abnormal forces. Non-working occlusal interferences (i.e. during excursive movements) are less common, although simultaneous working and non-working contacts are frequent. However, unless these features can be related to the signs or symptoms described in (a–c), occlusal treatment should not be contemplated, even as a prophylactic measure, since the periodontal tissues possess considerable powers of adaptation and the hazards of occlusal therapy are many.

Finally, there is no evidence that occlusal therapy, *per se*, can retard a destructive periodontal lesion and it should never be relied upon to achieve this. The purpose of periodontal care is to arrest, or at least retard connective tissue attachment loss, an inflammatory process which is *plaque induced.* Only *plaque control* can preserve periodontal attachment.

OCCLUSAL ADJUSTMENT

Occlusal adjustment for periodontal purposes refers to the process of reshaping the occluding surface to alter the magnitude, direction or distribution of forces on an individual tooth or group of teeth. This is usually achieved by grinding or sometimes by a restoration. Occlusal adjustment must be differentiated from the more elaborate process of occlusal equilibration, which refers to the alteration of the occlusal surfaces to provide stable, simultaneous, multiple, even contacts between opposing teeth.

Examples of Occlusal Adjustment

The centric interference. Premature contact(s) in the path of closure into centric occlusion, involving posterior teeth, may create an anterior adaptive path of closure, subjecting one or more of the upper incisor teeth to an anterior force (Fig. 15.1(a). The infrequent contacts during swallowing are unlikely to have any serious effect. If, however, there has been some destruction of the supporting tissue of an anterior tooth due to periodontal disease, there will be less resistance to the anterior force. If the patient is a bruxist or clenches his teeth habitually, the duration and intensity of the force will be greatly increased. The result may be anterior tooth migration or, if sufficient reciprocal force is exerted by the lower lip, the tooth will maintain its position in the arch but will become hypermobile.

In the case of anterior tooth migration, as the tooth is pushed forwards, there is usually further eruption of the upper and sometimes also the lower incisors. Thus, lower incisor contact with the upper incisor is maintained and the anterior migration continues. When confronted with this, there should be a careful examination of the occlusion to establish whether occlusal adjustment should be carried out. By appropriate grinding of posterior teeth in the retruded contact position of the mandible, it is sometimes possible to reposition the mandible and provide stable occlusal contacts distal to the habitual intercuspal position (Fig. 15.1(b)). Although this may appear to be a straightforward procedure when seen diagrammatically as in Figure 15.1, it must

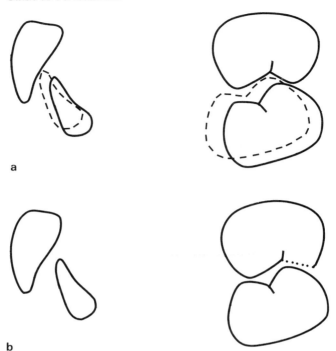

Fig. 15.1   *Elimination of a centric interference. (a) In the retruded position, a premature contact would occur (continuous line). The patient adopts an anterior path of closure to reach the intercuspal position (broken line), the lower incisor pushing forwards against the upper incisor. (b) The offending cusp of the upper molar is ground (dotted line), stabilising the mandible in a more distal position. The upper incisor may now be retracted.*

be emphasised that it is usually a time-consuming process and may involve the undesirable destruction of large amounts of tooth enamel from every posterior tooth.

The eccentric interference. A posterior tooth which is affected by plaque-induced periodontal disease, and therefore by destruction of supporting tissue, may become mobile, particularly if the tooth is 'rocked' in its socket during excursive movements. A reduction of mobility (if desired) may be achieved by grinding the upper buccal and lower lingual cusps, thus reducing lateral forces on the teeth while maintaining functional contacts around centric occlusion (Fig. 15.2). This procedure can be carried out with relative ease so that splints are rarely required for stabilisation of posterior teeth. However, if a group of teeth

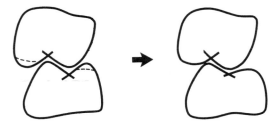

Fig. 15.2 *Grinding (broken line) to limit functional contacts in right lateral excursion. Note that maximum contact is maintained around centric occlusion.*

are equally mobile, any reduction of lateral stress on any one tooth will be offset by additional stress upon the remaining teeth, which may become increasingly mobile.

Anterior teeth, which are affected by loss of periodontal support and which have become mobile, are rarely amenable to occlusal adjustment. If the incisal edge of a lower anterior tooth is ground off to eliminate a protrusive interference, this will cause loss of contact in centric occlusion and invite over-eruption of the lower incisor to re-establish its previous unsatisfactory occlusal relationship with its opponent in the upper arch. Protrusive interferences, therefore, can be eliminated and stable occlusal relationships produced only by grinding the palatal slopes and incisal edges of upper incisors and canines, and this would have unwelcome aesthetic effects. This is particularly true in cases of increased overbite. Splinting is often, therefore, a more appropriate means of occlusal therapy for anterior teeth.

The plunger cusp. Food impaction is often associated with a 'plunger' cusp mechanism. This is usually amenable to occlusal adjustment (Fig. 15.3) and restoration of the open contact area.

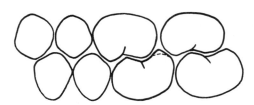

Fig. 15.3 *The plunger cusp mechanism, causing food impaction between |6 and |7, can be eliminated by grinding along the dotted line.*

SPLINTING

Splinting is the procedure by which a tooth's resistance to an applied force is increased by joining it to a neighbouring tooth or teeth. Splints may be classified as temporary or permanent, fixed or removable.

Like occlusal adjustment, splints are used less frequently nowadays, not only because fewer indications are recognised, but also because of their harmful effects: sound tooth substance may have to be destroyed; plaque control may be impaired; and aesthetics may be unsatisfactory. The rationale of splinting is described by Lindhe and Nyman (1977). Splints are used in periodontics principally to stabilise anterior teeth which are subject to migration, or to retain anterior teeth which have been realigned. They may also be used to stabilise teeth which are so mobile that they interfere with patient comfort especially during mastication. There is a wide variety of splints in current use. A few of the more useful types are described below.

The Composite Resin-retained Splint

Composite resin alone lacks sufficient transverse strength to splint mobile teeth, unless used in great bulk. However, it may be used as a cementing medium for the 'Rochette' or 'Maryland' splints. These comprise custom-made cast bars in non-precious alloy, fitting against the lingual surfaces of teeth. The composite cement engages tooth enamel on one side and, on the other, either countersunk perforations in the bar (Rochette technique) (Fig. 15.4) or an electrolytically etched metal fitting surface (Maryland technique). The appropriate clinical and technical procedures have been described by Tay and Shaw (1979) and by Wood (1982).

These techiques are particularly applicable to lower anterior teeth where it is now rarely necessary to advocate a more elaborate method. They are also frequently suitable for upper anterior teeth, but only where occlusal relationships will accommodate the necessary thickness of metal.

Published studies on the long-term success rates of composite resin-retained splints are few, but anecdotal evidence suggests that failure of Rochette and Maryland splints is not uncommon. Some consideration should, therfore, be given to the ease of repair of different types of splint. In this respect, the multistrand

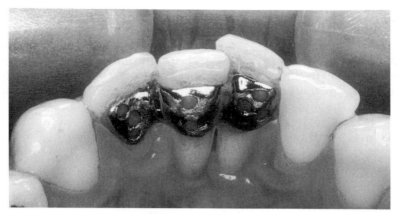

Fig. 15.4   *Mirror view of lower anterior teeth showing a 'Rochette' splint* in situ *stabilising the hypermobile* $\overline{11}$.

wire splint can be recommended. This consists of a spiral wire adapted to the lingual tooth surfaces on a plaster model, transferred to the mouth and cemented to the cingulum region of each tooth. Each tooth retains slight independent mobility. These splints are inexpensive to fabricate and easy to repair. The composite resin does not cover a large expanse of lingual tooth surface and can be utilised in the upper anterior region in cases of 'normal' as well as 'incomplete' overbite.

The Full-coverage Splint

This is useful where an increased overbite exists, preventing the construction of an upper resin-retained splint. It is also the technique of choice for splinting heavily restored or otherwise unsightly teeth. Serious consideration, however, should be given to avoiding a full-coverage splint when teeth are intact, since large amounts of tooth substance must be destroyed to accommodate metal and porcelain and there is a significant risk of pulpal damage due to the technical difficulty of making multiple parallel preparations.

The Removable Acrylic Occlusal Splint (Bite Plane)

In cases which are unsuitable for either of the foregoing methods, the construction of an acrylic occlusal splint as a night-guard appliance may be considered. This consists simply of an acrylic splint with incisor edge cover, retained by Adams cribs on molar teeth. It is worn at night to stabilise teeth which during the day possess a potential to drift forwards. This type of splint is also useful where large spaces are present between upper incisors, preventing the construction of an aesthetically acceptable fixed splint.

These splints, however, tend to become unhygienic and suffer occlusal wear and need to be replaced periodically.

The Removable Partial Denture

In the management of tooth mobility and migration, the advantage of a removable partial denture is often limited to its effect in redistributing masticatory load rather than to any effect of the rigid denture base components. As a general rule, upper anterior teeth are difficult to stabilise with a partial denture, since it is impractical to place a metal clasp on their labial surfaces. There is, however, at least one exception—the 'swinglock' partial denture, which is used to restore missing posterior teeth and carries a hinged labial 'locking' bar within the labial vestibule to which may be added an acrylic 'gingival' veneer. This labial flange may be used, not only as a splint, but also to mask the enlarged interdental spaces which are frequently present between teeth which have received periodontal treatment.

In the lower arch, the swinglock denture may be employed without its acrylic veneer whilst retaining its splinting effect, since there are metal struts leading from the labial connecting bar to the necks of the teeth. Such a design minimises plaque accumulation.

ANTERIOR TOOTH MIGRATION

Mention has been made already in this and other chapters of various aspects of anterior tooth migration. The management of anterior tooth migration embraces many aspects of occlusal therapy and will now be considered in more detail.

Anterior tooth migration is a common complaint of patients presenting with periodontal disease. Drifting may occur at a rate consistent with the rate of periodontal deterioration. Alternatively it may be a sequel to tooth loss or the adoption of a parafunctional habit. Patients' thresholds of perception of changes in anterior tooth position and their degree of anxiety about them vary widely, and migration may be noted before significant increase in tooth mobility.

Aetiology

The following is a list of common aetiological factors:

a)   marginal periodontitis;
b)   periapical osteitis;
c)   loss of adjacent teeth;
d)   loss of posterior teeth with distal drift of part of the anterior segment.
e)   centric interferences: either a premature contact between the affected anterior tooth and its opponent or, more commonly, a posterior deflective contact creating an anterior path of closure;
f)   protrusive interferences;
g)   parafunctional habits such as lip biting, nail biting, pipe smoking and playing a wind instrument.

Treatment

The first priority in treatment is the removal of aetiological factors as far as possible before corrective treatment is attempted. The list of possible management options will, therefore, include:

a)   periodontal and endodontic treatment;
b)   elimination of parafunctional habits;
c)   monitoring tooth positions with study casts;
d)   occlusal adjustment;
e)   replacement of missing teeth;
f)   splinting in the new position;
g)   orthodontic realignment and splinting;
h)   repositioning by crown construction;
i)   composite augmentation to reduce spaces;
j)   extraction and prosthesis.

The initial aim of periodontal therapy will be the establishment of periodontal health with the arrest of marginal bone loss. Where infrabony pockets are present, bone-fill may be achieved by open-flap curettage. Endodontic treatment, where required, should improve periapical support.

These measures alone may be sufficient to achieve tooth stability and reduce the risk of further migration. Therefore, if the new tooth position is acceptable to the patient, reference casts may be obtained to monitor tooth position. Where doubt persists concerning tooth stability, splinting may be employed as described earlier in this chapter, although it may be advisable to realign the tooth first.

Where the position of the migrated tooth is cosmetically unacceptable, orthodontic treatment should be considered, and will be simply accomplished so long as space is available for realignment. Frequently, however, upper anterior tooth migration is accompanied by anterior migration of lower teeth and/or by extrusion of the migrated teeth or their opponents. Orthodontic therapy will then involve appliance therapy in both arches and/or intrusion of over-erupted teeth. Very occasionally, it may be possible to create space for retraction of upper anterior teeth by occlusal adjustment to stabilise the mandible in a more distal occlusal position. This, of course, will be possible only where there is a posterior deflective contact.

After realignment, permanent splinting is almost always necessary and an acceptable means by which this may be achieved should be determined before orthodontic therapy commences.

Tooth realignment, by means of artificial crowns on realigned posts and cores following endodontic treatment, is usually only possible where the desired anterior tooth position has not been invaded by lower anterior teeth. It is essential to check that a stable position can be found for the new crowns, preferably by the use of mounted diagnostic casts. If a stable position cannot be found, some means of permanent retention will be necessary.

DEEP TRAUMATIC OVERBITE

Clinical Features
(Fig. 15.5)

The development of incisor tooth relationships depends on the skeletal form and on incisor inclination which itself may be influenced by tongue and lip activity. Deep overbite may also

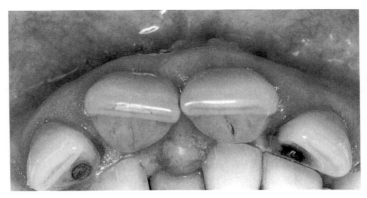

Fig. 15.5 *Deep traumatic overbite.*

arise in a previously normal occlusion affected by anterior tooth migration and over-eruption. The likelihood of gingival trauma occurring is increased by loss of posterior support and by clenching or grinding habits. Food impaction is a frequent source of acute pain and swelling. Periodontitis, therefore, becomes established and further loss of periodontal support may occur through gingival recession and recurrent periodontal abscesses.

Treatment

Successful treatment is dependent not only on the relief of trauma and control of infection but also on the establishment of stable centric contacts.

The first treatment option in young patients with traumatic overbite should be orthodontic therapy, perhaps involving intrusion of the anterior teeth or extrusion of the posterior teeth, uprighting of tilted incisors and reduction of overjet. Extreme cases may benefit from orthognathic surgery.

Many adults with deep overbite have excellent occlusal function without trauma and should not normally be offered treatment prophylactically. If trauma has occurred, it may be relieved by grinding the incisal edges of impinging incisors or by increasing the vertical dimension of occlusion, making sure that appropriate measures are undertaken to prevent further incisor extrusion. Very occasionally, if there is an associated posterior centric interference with an anterior adaptive path of closure, occlusal adjustment may be attempted to reposition the mandible distally, as described above.

Whatever methods are used to eliminate the impinging overbite, among those described above, it is *imperative* that steps are also taken to prevent incisor over-eruption. The problem of further extrusion is usually limited to the lower incisors since the upper incisors are prevented from over-eruption by the muscle tone of the lower lip, except where there is a very high lip line as in some Angle Class II Division 2 malocclusions. Stability of the lower incisors is most usually achieved by fitting, as a night-guard, an upper acrylic splint with an anterior bite plane to occlude against lower incisors. If there are missing teeth, the metal base of an upper partial denture can be designed to occlude against the lower incisors or else the lingual plate connector of a lower partial denture can be carried on to the incisal edges. Partial dentures, can, if necessary, be constructed with posterior onlays where reduction of a lower incisor is impracticable. Another means of stabilising shortened lower incisors involves the use of a resin-retained splint extending backwards in the arch until teeth with stable centric contacts are included.

Conclusion

Deep traumatic overbite is a multidisciplinary problem. It may occur in patients with good plaque control and good gingival conditions as well as in patients with poor plaque control and gingivitis. In theory, healthy gingiva should be more resistant to trauma and food impaction than diseased gingiva. Therefore, the maintenance of good oral hygiene and good periodontal conditions may help to reduce the incidence of this form of occlusal trauma.

REFERENCES

Lindhe J., Nyman S. (1977). The role of occlusion in periodontal disease and the biologic rationale for splinting in treatment of periodontitis. *Oral Sciences Reviews*; **10**: 11–43.

Ramfjord S. P., Ash M. M., Jr. (1983). *Occlusion*. Philadelphia: W. B. Saunders.

Tay W. M., Shaw M. J. (1979). The Rochette adhesive bridge. *Dental Update*; **6**: 153–7.

Wise M. D. (1986). *Occlusion and Restorative Dentistry for the General Practitioner*, 2nd edn. London: British Dental Association.

Wood M. (1982). Etched casting resin bonded retainers: an improved technique for periodontal splinting. *International Journal of Periodontics and Restorative Dentistry*; 2: 9–26.

FURTHER READING

Akerley W. B. (1977). Prosthodontic treatment of traumatic overlap of the anterior teeth. *Journal of Prosthetic Dentistry*; **38**: 26–34.

Becker A. (1987). Periodontal splinting with multistrand wire following orthodontic realignment of migrated teeth: report of 38 cases. *International Journal of Adult Orthodontics and Orthognathic Surgery*; **2**: 99–109.

Dawson P. E. (1974). Solving deep overbite problems. In *Evaluation, diagnosis and treatment of occlusal problems*. Ch. 23. St. Louis: Mosby.

Polson A. (1980). Efficacy of occlusal adjustment in periodontal therapy. In *Efficacy of Treatment Procedures in Periodontics*. (Shanley D. ed.) p. 245. Chicago: Quintessence.

Watkinson A. C., Hathorn I. S. (1986). Occlusion in the aetiology and management of upper anterior tooth migration. *Restorative Dentistry*; **2**: 56–61.

Chapter 16

Recall Maintenance

Since the bacteria causing periodontal disease belong to the indigenous flora, they will persist in the mouth even after the establishment of complete periodontal health. Furthermore, innumerable studies have shown that the great majority of patients, having completed a course of periodontal treatment, will thereafter exhibit a decline in plaque control and a recurrence of gingivitis and periodontal destruction, unless they are subjected to a programme of maintenance care.

The reasons for this breakdown in plaque control are many: they include a failure of motivation, failure to remember oral hygiene instructions and the accumulation of calculus deposits, providing a bed for plaque growth. Maintenance care, therefore, should include where necessary, remotivation, reinstruction and scaling and polishing, including subgingival scaling if appropriate.

OBJECTIVES OF MAINTENANCE CARE

The recall programme should be designed to maintain the degree of periodontal health which was achieved during the treatment phase and, at the same time, maintain attachment levels. The objectives of the maintenance phase will, therefore, depend on the success of the treatment phase.

Optimum periodontal health is recognised by the absence of bleeding on probing and this is usually accompanied by resistance to the probing force and, therefore, by shallow probing depths. It must be remembered, however, that treatment may have been concluded without achieving perfect periodontal health. The level of home care, during treatment, may not have been compatible with gingival health or the success of professional care may have been limited by subgingival restorations, age, infirmity or lack of availability for treatment. Nevertheless, in most of these cases, a measure of improvement will have been obtained. This may be recognised by the patient as a reduction in halitosis, bad taste or bleeding when brushing. The operator may note less bleeding on probing, a reduction in probing depths and a reduction in tooth mobility—all signs of an improved prognosis.

Maintenance care is necessary for all patients: those who have been rendered free of periodontal disease and those in whom the inflammatory process has been contained rather than eradicated. These two groups of patients will require different maintenance regimes.

FREQUENCY OF RECALL VISITS

Where absolute periodontal health has not been achieved by treatment, patients should be recalled at intervals of about three months. Where absolute periodontal health has been achieved, the recall intervals should be tailored to suit individual needs. Patients who have been subjected to periodontal surgery and who are using chlorhexidine mouthwash during the immediate postoperative period should be re-examined three or four weeks after stopping the mouthwash to make sure that their plaque control methods are adequate to cope with the altered gingival architecture. Recall intervals should be gradually increased, depending on the patient's ability to sustain motivation and the rapidity with which calculus accumulates. It is rarely practicable to provide recall prophylaxis at less than three-month intervals and probably unwise to allow the interval to exceed one year. If, at any recall visit, there is evidence of periodontal breakdown, the recall frequency should be increased.

PRACTICAL RECALL PROCEDURES

Patients with Healthy Periodontal Tissue

Assuming that tooth surface débridement has been carried out adequately during the treatment phase, the critical factor determining the long-term success of periodontal therapy is the standard of self-performed plaque control practised by the patient on a daily basis. Recall visits are a means of encouraging the patient to evaluate and, if necessary, adjust tooth-cleaning techniques. Furthermore, at sites of recurrent periodontitis, the clinician will have the opportunity to rescue the situation by subgingival instrumentation before deep-seated disease becomes re-established.

When the maintenance programme and the patient's attention to oral hygiene is sufficient to maintain a physiological gingival sulcus, attachment loss will not occur and there is little point, therefore, in monitoring attachment levels; attachment loss is difficult and time consuming to measure since it involves identification of the amelocemental junction as well as the base of the pocket.

The following protocol is suggested for recall visits.

a)   Initial discussion with the patient to identify new or recurrent oral problems.
b)   Identification of sites of supragingival plaque accumulation and gingivitis. Reinforcement of oral hygiene procedures.
c)   Identification and removal of supragingival calculus.
d)   Identification of pathological pockets. Subgingival scaling and root planing as necessary.
e)   Assessment of restorations, removal of overhangs, etc.
f)   Assessment of mobility levels and of teeth subject to migration. Stabilisation procedures, if necessary.
g)   Polishing all accessible surfaces.
h)   Treatment of sensitive teeth.
i)   Decision on timing of next recall appointment.

Patients with Persistent Disease

Maintenance care for these patients takes the form of an extension of the treatment phase, with repeated scaling and reinforced oral hygiene instruction to maintain the level of improvement achieved during treatment or, more realistically, to retard further deterioration. A major problem is how to administer the maintenance care to greatest effect in one visit (if possible) when multiple deep pockets are present and oral hygiene is unsatisfactory. The standard routine described above to maintain periodontal health is not applicable to this type of patient. Instead, the clinician must devise an individual strategy to deal with each patient with the following considerations in mind.

Ideally, one would choose to target those pathological pockets where further attachment loss is imminent. Unfortunately, there are no clinical or microbiological tests currently available which can forecast disease activity.

There is little point in wasting time by keeping a record of attachment levels with the intention of identifying those sites which have recently suffered loss of attachment. Even if it were possible to measure attachment loss quickly and accurately, this would serve little purpose. Research has shown that sites which have recently suffered attachment loss do not present a greater risk of further attachment loss than previously stable sites.

Not all teeth are of equal value. Some are of greater strategic importance than others. Anterior and premolar teeth usually have a greater treatment priority than molars but a single standing molar may be useful as a bridge or partial-denture abutment.

Removal of supragingival calculus can be carried out quickly and atraumatically and should facilitate daily personal oral hygiene. In addition, the patient's impression of oral cleanliness may motivate him to a better standard of home care.

At sites of persistent plaque accumulation, subgingival instrumentation cannot be fully effective but may produce a temporary remission. Experiments have shown that several months may elapse before the main periodontal pathogens are re-established in the proportions observed prior to débridement. This would account for the research finding that regularly repeated débridement in patients with inadequate oral hygiene will reduce the rate of overall attachment loss. With a large number of pathological pockets in one mouth, however, the clinician may be forced to decide which sites justify most attention. In this respect, preservation of remaining attachment has an added significance for teeth of strategic importance already affected by advanced attachment loss. Débridement of very deep pockets, however, particularly those with associated furcation lesions, may not be very effective and there is always the risk of precipitating a periodontal abscess.

In conclusion, there is a serious lack of scientific knowledge on suitable maintenance regimes for patients whose standards of plaque control are not consistent with periodontal health. Until such data are forthcoming, maintenance care for these individuals will remain empirical.

FURTHER READING

Axelsson P., Lindhe J. (1981). The significance of maintenance care in the treatment of periodontal disease. *Journal of Clinical Periodontology*; **8**: 281–94.

Hirschfeld L., Wasserman B. (1978). A long-term survey of tooth loss in 600 treated periodontal patients. *Journal of Periodontology*; **49**: 225–37.

Lindhe J., Nyman S. (1984). Long-term maintenance of patients treated for advanced periodontal disease. *Journal of Clinical Periodontology*; **11**: 504–15.

Lindhe J., Westfelt E., Nyman S., Socransky S. S., Haffajee A. D. (1984). Long term effect of surgical/non-surgical treatment of periodontal disease. *Journal of Clinical Periodontology*; **11**: 448–58.

Ramfjord S. P. (1987). Maintenance care for treated periodontitis patients. *Journal of Clinical Periodontology*; **14**: 433–8.

Shick R. A. (1981). Maintenance phase of periodontal therapy. *Journal of Periodontology*; **52**: 576–83.

Chapter 17

Periodontal Aspects of Restorative Dentistry

Restorations and prostheses should be designed not only to minimise plaque accumulation in the proximity of the marginal periodontal tissues but also to avoid physical injury to the gingiva and periodontal membrane. This chapter is devoted to a consideration of gingival-margin–restoration relationships and to discussion of the support potential of the reduced periodontium. The reader is referred to the listed texts for further information on the inter-relationship of periodontal disease and restorative dentistry.

NATURAL HISTORY OF PROXIMAL AND CERVICAL CARIES

The usual site of caries attack on smooth surfaces is immediately coronal to the gingival margin (Fig. 17.1(a)), assuming that normal gingival contours are present. This applies both to proximal surface lesions and to the cervical region of buccal and lingual surfaces. Although the enamel lesion may taper towards the amelodentinal junction, when that junction is reached, there is considerable spread (Fig. 17.1(a)) to involve a much larger area of dentine. The apical extension of the dentine lesion is frequently subgingival, and may even reach the level of the alveolar crest. Subgingivally, the enamel overlying the dentine may remain intact and the integrity of the dentogingival junction may not be affected by the carious process. In order to restore such a carious lesion, however, some destruction of the subgingival enamel is inevitable and, with it, destruction of the epithelial attachment (Fig. 17.1(b)).

Whatever restoration is chosen, be it gold, porcelain, amalgam or composite, the prospect of epithelial attachment to the restoration would appear to be remote, and a pocket is formed to the apical extent of the restoration. Thus, the epithelial barrier, which normally prevents access by oral bacteria to the

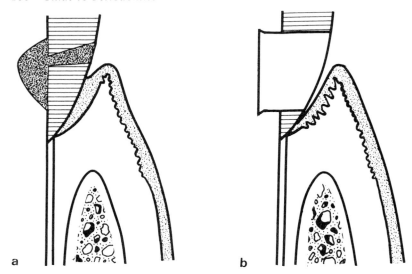

Fig. 17.1   *Restoration of cervical caries.* (a) *Caries at the gingival margin extending into dentine.* (b) *The restoration extending subgingivally with pocket formation.*

subgingival environment, is lost, making colonisation of the subgingival restoration surface inevitable. It is well established that bacterial adhesion to restoration surfaces is greater than to intact tooth substance, mainly because of differences in surface energy. Furthermore, once established, complete removal of bacterial plaque from a comparatively rough restoration surface with a marginal imperfection at the tooth–restoration interface is virtually impossible.

All subgingival restorations, therefore, even those judged to be clinically satisfactory, are likely to cause gingivitis of some degree, together with a gingival or periodontal pocket which will extend at least to the apical margin of the restoration. The periodontal condition, will, of course, be further prejudiced by restorations which are not satisfactory.

APPROACHES TO THE RESTORATION OF PROXIMAL AND CERVICAL CARIES

With the above in mind, it need hardly be stated that cavity preparation should not extend subgingivally except, where necessary, to excavate caries and remove seriously undermined enamel. This rule, however, will require some modification in the case of an anterior jacket crown restoration (*see below*).

Amalgam Restorations

Amalgam restorations should be adequately condensed to reduce surface imperfections. A matrix should be used to contain the amalgam in a Class II cavity. The matrix should be wedged and properly contoured to the outline of the enamel margin of the cervical floor. However, in spite of the universal acceptance of matrices for this purpose, a good cervical fit is often difficult to achieve where the cervical floor is at or below the gingival level (Fig. 17.2), where the proximal surface is concave (Fig. 17.3), or where the matrix tends to ride off the tooth as it is tightened. Textbooks of operative dentistry should be consulted for methods which overcome these difficulties, although much will

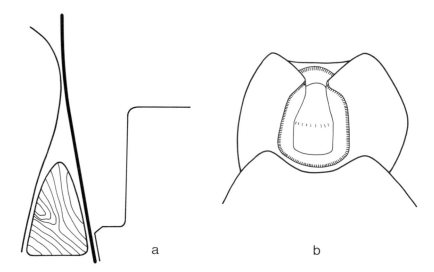

a   b

Fig. 17.2   *Relationship of the cervical wedge to the cavity margin.* (a) *Proper position of the wedge supporting the matrix apical to the cavity margin, achievable only by compressing the interdental gingiva.* (b) *The cervical margin lies within the interdental gingival depression, a normal feature in posterior tooth segments; the wedge must displace the buccal and lingual papillae apically to be located in its proper position, or else electrosurgical removal of these papillae may have to be considered.*

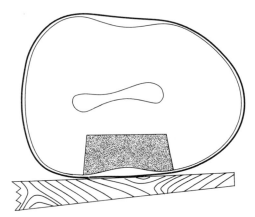

Fig. 17.3 *Section through a Class II cavity at the level of the cervical floor showing how the wedge fails to adapt the matrix to the cavity margin when a proximal furrow is present.*

ultimately depend on improvisation and the ingenuity of the operator. The skill required to complete a satisfactory amalgam restoration is undoubtedly often underestimated. Failure to prevent cervical escape of amalgam necessitates immediate trimming using a fine probe before the alloy has set. If this trimming is postponed, to be attempted later with a finishing burr, there will be a risk of damage to the periodontium and tooth surface.

If, in spite of all precautions, an amalgam overhang is unavoidable and if it is inaccessible for trimming with a fine probe, an alternative restoration such as a gold inlay should be considered.

Composite Restorations

A wide range of composite filling and veneering materials is now available for restoration of anterior and posterior teeth.

In anterior teeth, the composite resin should be carefully adapted to the cavity using an appropriate matrix and any excess fractured off when set, to leave a good tooth–restoration junction. Bulky overhanging margins should be avoided since composite materials do not respond well to finishing procedures, the surface becoming rougher and more plaque-retentive. Cervical fit should be assessed with a sharp probe and dental floss before passing the restoration as satisfactory.

These observations apply equally to the use of posterior composite resins. While these newer materials have the advantages over amalgam of bonding to tooth substance, splinting cusps and better appearance, their use on approximal surfaces is still problematic. The use of a rubber dam is at least desirable, if not mandatory, for satisfactory control of moisture. Placement of a matrix which will prevent escape of composite resin cervically, yet allow construction of a satisfactory interdental contact area in a material less easily condensed than amalgam, is difficult. Failure to attend to these details may lead to cervical overhangs or deficiency, inadequate contact areas, or leakage due to inadequate bonding to enamel or dentine. The risk of plaque retention and food impaction is, thereby, increased. It is the authors' view that, in spite of many favourable properties, posterior composite resins are not yet suitable for *routine* use in place of amalgam.

PERIODONTAL CARE OF TEETH WITH SUBGINGIVAL RESTORATIONS

The majority of proximal surface restorations extend into a gingival or periodontal pocket. Many buccal or lingual surface restorations also finish subgingivally, although the tendency for gingival recession to occur on buccal surfaces will, in time, often lead to a supragingival margin. Effects of subgingival restorations on the periodontal tissues will depend to a large extent on the care taken to achieve an accurately fitting restoration, free from surface imperfections as far as possible. It must be emphasised, however, that even a perfectly formed restoration will, by retaining plaque subgingivally, cause some degree of gingivitis and may initiate a destructive periodontal lesion.

The harmful effects of a subgingival restoration can, to some extent, be mitigated by the daily use of dental floss interproximally within the pocket and employment of the Bass technique of intrasulcular brushing (*see* Fig. 8.1) for buccal and lingual surfaces. Ideally, surgical pocket elimination, leading to a physiological gingival sulcus apical to the cervical margin of the restoration, should be carried out. This, however, will be possible only if a deep pathological pocket exists where the alveolar bone margin is at least 4 mm apical to the restoration margin, or if the operator is prepared to sacrifice bone to achieve

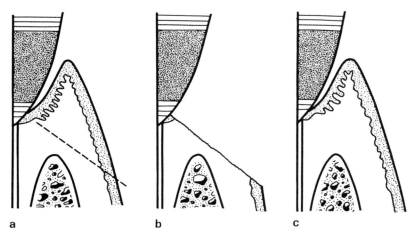

a   b   c

Fig. 17.4 *Gingivectomy and the subgingival restoration: restoration to bone magin distance < 4 mm. (a) The incision to the base of the pocket. (b) The wound with the exposed filling margin. (c) Months later, when gingival regeneration is complete, the restoration is once again subgingivally located with pocket formation.*

such a bone-margin–restoration relationship (Van der Velden, 1982). Figure 17.4 illustrates why a gingivectomy, for example, would be an inappropriate form of treatment to eliminate a pathological pocket which was associated with a deeply extended subgingival restoration. Removal of the gingival tissue to the base of the pocket (Fig. 17.4(b)) may initially expose the restoration margin in a supragingival position just coronal to the bone margin and this may facilitate impression procedures or accurate adjustment of subgingival margins. During soft-tissue repair, however, gingival tissue will tend to regain a physiological form (Van der Velden, 1982). When the final dimensions have been achieved, and this usually takes many months, the restoration will once again be subgingival. Gingival regeneration in this way will produce a marginal or papillary gingiva which extends about 4 mm coronal to the underlying crestal bone. While the removal of some marginal bone as well as gingiva would help to create a supragingival margin, such a step is rarely justifiable since many gingival pockets, even without treatment, will not progress to destructive periodontitis.

Figure 17.5 illustrates how a deeper pocket with a less extensive restoration may be managed by pocket elimination surgery such as the gingivectomy or apically repositioned flap.

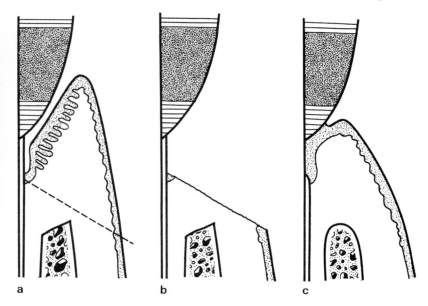

Fig. 17.5 *Gingivectomy and the subgingival restoration: restoration to bone margin distance > 4 mm. (a) The incision to the base of the pocket. (b) The wound with the exposed filling margin. (c) Months later, when gingival regeneration is complete, a physiological gingival sulcus has formed apical to the filling margin.*

Indeed, this situation is one of the indications for pocket elimination surgery (*see* Chapter 10).

During routine periodontal examination, the periodontal tissue adjacent to subgingivally extended fillings should be carefully appraised. Gingivitis will usually be observed, although in mild cases this may be evident only by a tendency to bleed on probing. Probing depths should be noted and the distance between the cervical margin of the restoration and the alveolar bone margin should be gauged by probing and by scrutiny of the radiographs. This is often difficult, for it must be remembered that the probe tip will probably not reach the bone margin, and radiographs must be taken with the x-ray beam perpendicular to the long axis of the tooth to give a true image which does not exaggerate the proximity of the restoration margin to the bone.

Where the restoration–bone-margin distance is judged to be 4 mm or more, and the patient can achieve a high standard of personal oral hygiene, periodontal surgery should be successful in eliminating the pocket and placing the restoration margin in a supragingival position.

Where the restoration–bone-margin distance is less than 4 mm, surgery will not usually be worthwhile for reasons already explained, unless the objective is to provide access for trimming and polishing of overhanging margins. Pathological pockets will usually persist and the dentist's responsibility will lie in periodic re-examination, in instituting a programme of regular subgingival débridement, perhaps at three-month intervals, and in making sure the patient receives appropriate oral hygiene instruction and motivation. If, at re-examination, probing depths have increased or radiographic evidence of further bone destruction is present, increasing the restoration–bone-margin distance, surgical intervention should be considered to locate the restoration margin in a supragingival position.

CROWN MARGINS

The case for a *supragingival* margin in the restoration of carious teeth clearly applies also in crown preparation. It has been argued that subgingival tooth preparation is necessary to create long axial walls for adequate retention. Aids to retention, however, such as steps, posts, pins, grooves or boxes should be considered first. Once a retentive preparation has been created supragingivally, impression procedures, temporary crown provision and final cementation will all be greatly simplified. The marginal seal may be inspected without difficulty, a factor of special importance for bridge retainers, which may undergo cementation failure while remaining *in situ*, attached to other parts of the bridge.

Whenever possible, therefore, all crown restorations should be designed with a supragingival margin—with the single possible exception of upper anterior and premolar crowns, where it is desirable, for aesthetic reasons, to conceal the labial margin within the gingival sulcus (Fig. 17.6). Provided the preparation extends no more than 0·5 mm apical to the gingival crest (i.e. no deeper than the base of the histological sulcus), little harm will result, although a mild gingivitis is virtually inevitable. On the other hand, deliberate subgingival extension beyond the base of the sulcus with disruption of the epithelial attachment should be

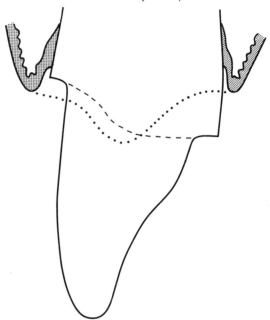

Fig. 17.6   *Sagittal section through an anterior jacket crown preparation. The buccal finishing line is located within the gingival sulcus. The lingual finishing line is located in a supragingival position. Outside the plane of section, the dotted line represents the outline of the interdental gingival margin and the broken line represents the interdental cervical margin of the crown preparation.*

condemned. This will lead to subgingival plaque accumulation and gingivitis, possibly to be followed by periodontitis and gingival recession. Indeed, it is confirmed in a number of research reports that deeply placed subgingival margins on labial tooth aspects may promote gingival recession and so defeat their original purpose of aesthetic restoration.

Although crown construction is always easier when carried out wholly on the visible tooth surface, the operative work is unlikely to be seriously compromised by a subgingival extension of up to 0·5 mm. The result should be an accurately fitting crown with a highly polished or glazed surface located at the front of the mouth, where the patient has optimum access for oral hygiene and should be able to clean the crown margin with an intrasulcular technique such as the Bass method. Subgingival placement of anterior jacket crown margins should not, however, extend to the proximal or palatal aspects, where a supragingival finishing line is desirable for minimal interference with gingival health (Fig. 17.6).

When periodontal surgery is planned, definitive anterior crown\preparation should be delayed for at least 20 weeks after surgery until the position of the gingival crest is stable (Wise, 1985).

SUPPORT POTENTIAL OF THE REDUCED PERIODONTIUM

Definition

In this section 'reduced periodontium' refers to a situation where there is a marked reduction in number of teeth or severe attachment loss, thereby reducing the periodontal support available for a partial prosthesis.

Fixed or Removable?

In general, a fixed bridge is preferable to a removable partial denture. It is less obtrusive, causes less enhancement of plaque accumulation and is, therefore, less likely to promote periodontal disease. On the other hand, more clinical and technical expertise is required, and the cost implications are greater.

There has been a tendency in the past to reserve bridgework for short spans where the abutment teeth have good periodontal support and to construct removable partial dentures for patients whose abutment teeth are few in number or are poorly supported. However, the shortcomings of partial dentures are even more obvious in cases of reduced periodontal support. Where edentulous free-end saddle areas or other long spans exist, flexure or tilting of the denture base is likely. This may result in gingival and mucosal trauma. Soft-tissue trauma may also result from denture movement as teeth, already mobile, are rocked by denture components such as clasp arms and connectors. In theory, this should not occur if proper reciprocation is employed, but in practice a period of periodontal 'adaptation' often follows the insertion of a new partial denture, at the end of which abutment teeth may be so mobile that retention and support are compromised and gingival trauma arises as a result of movement of the denture base in function. This problem may be overcome by provision of fixed bridgework of cross-arch design.

Advantages of Bridgework

Although the above-mentioned drawbacks of partial dentures are well recognised and fully acknowledged, prosthodontists have felt constrained by 'Ante's Law' from providing fixed bridgework in cases of reduced periodontal support. Ante proposed that in a fixed bridge the root surface area of the abutment teeth should be equal to or greater than the root surface area of the teeth to be replaced by pontics. While this may be considered safe advice, there is no doubt that such a rigid formula places considerable constraints on abutment selection. At the other extreme, Nyman and Ericsson (1982) have shown that, provided healthy periodontal conditions are maintained, satisfactory function can be achieved with bridges which rely on markedly reduced periodontal support—as little as 16% of the presumed root surface area of the teeth replaced by pontics. Thus, bridgework is possible and indeed preferable even for patients with reduced periodontal support. This is especially so when there is significant tooth mobility, since the greater rigidity of the fixed reconstruction provides a more favourable distribution of masticatory function to the remaining periodontium.

Notwithstanding the clinical and technical difficulties of fixed bridgework in general, the *reduced* periodontium may afford certain advantages to the clinician and technician. Increased clinical crown length should allow preparation of abutments with excellent retention form and, if aesthetics allow, supragingival margins. Moreover, increased vertical space will be available (owing to alveolar bone loss) to construct components of sufficient dimension to resist the deformation which can lead to fracture of metal, porcelain or cement lute. Finally, it should be noted that mechanoreceptors within the periodontal membrane restrict, by feedback, the amount of force generated by the muscles of mastication, and thereby, limit the load on the bridge.

Concluding Remarks

It is, of course, essential that advanced periodontal disease is treated successfully before a complex and costly fixed prosthesis is provided. If periodontal health cannot be achieved and advanced periodontitis persists, the prognosis for the dentition will be poor, regardless of the method chosen for tooth replacement. Then economic factors will usually dictate provision of a removable prosthesis. When the prognosis is particularly poor, this should be regarded as a transitional denture, that is, a partial denture which is provided as part of the planned transition to a complete denture.

REFERENCES

Nyman S., Ericsson I. (1982). The capacity of reduced periodontal tissues to support fixed bridgework. *Journal of Clinical Periodontology*; **9**: 409–14.

Van der Velden U. (1982). Regeneration of the interdental soft tissues following denudation procedures. *Journal of Clinical Periodontology*; **9**: 455–9.

Wise M. D. (1985). Stability of gingival crest after surgery and before anterior crown placement. *Journal of Prosthetic Dentistry*; **53**: 20–3.

FURTHER READING

Jenkins W. M. M. (1981). Periodontal aspects of restorative dentistry—Part 1. *Dental Update*; **8**: 489–94.

Jenkins W. M. M. (1981). Periodontal aspects of restorative dentistry—Part 2. *Dental Update*; **8**: 569–77.

Leon A. R. (1977). The periodontium and restorative procedures. *Journal of Oral Rehabilitation*; **4**: 105–18.

Midda M., Watkinson A. C. (1980). The planning of restorative treatment. *Dental Update*; **7**: 409–16.

Nyman S., Lindhe J. (1979). A longitudinal study of combined periodontal and prosthetic treatment of patients with advanced periodontal disease. *Journal of Periodontology*; **50**: 163–9.

Ramfjord S. P., Ash M., Jr. (1979). Periodontal considerations in restorative and other aspects of dentistry. In *Periodontology and Periodontics*. p. 675. Eastbourne: W. B. Saunders.

Valderhaug J. (1980). Periodontal conditions following the insertion of fixed prostheses: a 10 year follow-up study. *International Dental Journal*; **30**: 296–304.

Chapter 18

Acute Conditions

ACUTE NECROTISING ULCERATIVE GINGIVITIS

Acute necrotising ulcerative gingivitis (ANUG) has been known by a variety of names including Vincent's infection, trench mouth, acute fuso-spirochaetal gingivitis and acute ulceromembranous gingivitis.

Clinical Presentation

Acute necrotising ulcerative gingivitis produces characteristic signs and symptoms, which usually make diagnosis relatively easy. It is a disease of sudden onset.

Inflammation. The gingivae become red and shiny and bleed easily.

Ulceration. As the name suggests this is the most characteristic feature of the disease. Classically, the ulcers form first on interdental papillae. With increasing severity, they spread to involve the marginal gingiva and, ultimately, in some untreated cases, the attached gingiva. The ulcers are extremely painful, a fact which may limit the amount of treatment which can be given at the initial visit. They are ragged in outline and are covered with a so-called 'pseudomembranous' slough (hence the name 'ulceromembranous gingivitis'). The slough consists of infected necrotic tissue and can be wiped off the surface of the ulcer, leaving a raw, bleeding, painful area. The condition is very destructive (hence 'necrotising gingivitis') and the interdental papilla may acquire a typical 'punched-out' appearance. If inadequately treated, the characteristic deformity may be evident for many years.

Halitosis. In most cases of ANUG there is a distinctive 'foetor oris'. The patient may also complain of an unpleasant or metallic taste.

Systemic effects. There is usually a degree of submental or submandibular lymphadenitis. In the more severe cases, there may be some cervical lymphadenitis, but systemic disturbance, if any, is mild.

Pain. As noted already, pain and extreme tenderness, even to gentle probing, are common and are important diagnostic signs in incipient ANUG, which may otherwise resemble chronic gingivitis.

Occurrence. Acute necrotising ulcerative gingivitis tends to occur in the second and third decades of life, the great majority of patients being between the ages of 18 and 26 years. It is rare in young children, the middle aged and elderly. The incidence of the disease is roughly equal in males and females.

Aetiology

The aetiology of ANUG is not entirely understood. It is considered to be a fuso-spirochaetal infection of gingival tissue which, for reasons unknown, has lowered resistance to infection. The following appear to be the most significant aetiological factors.

Inadequate oral hygiene. The overwhelming majority of ANUG cases occur in neglected mouths with inadequate plaque control. In a very few cases, however, areas of localised plaque retention may be present in an otherwise clean mouth. In such cases, the condition may be restricted to these zones. This would explain the common observation of ANUG around partially erupted lower wisdom teeth and imbricated incisors.

Fuso-spirochaetal complex. When the slough is wiped from the surface of the ulcers, and is examined microscopically, an overgrowth of various micro-organisms is observed, among which spirochaetes and fusiform bacilli are prominent. This is termed the fuso-spirochaetal complex and is the reason for the term 'fuso-spirochaetal gingivitis'. These organisms may even be seen invading the superficial layers of inflamed gingiva beneath the pseudomembrane. The consistent observation that these organisms are present in the slough led to the early supposition that they were the causative agents and that ANUG was contagious. However, attempts to reproduce the disease in healthy volunteers by transfer of fuso-spirochaetal organisms have failed. Spirochaetes and fusiforms belong to the indigenous flora and are present in mature plaque, but the reason for their apparent overgrowth in ANUG is not clear. In a recent bacteriological study of ANUG which implicated *Bacteroides melaninogenicus* ssp., *intermedius*, along with the fuso-spirochaetal complex, the following proposal was made: '. . .

these particular anaerobic species gained ascendency in the plaque as a result of being selected through the availability of host-derived nutrients in individuals who had undergone certain physiological and psychological stresses' (Loesche *et al.*, 1982).

Smoking. Acute necrotising ulcerative gingivitis is much more common amongst smokers than non-smokers. The reason for this observation is not entirely understood, but a number of explanations have been put forward, such as poorer plaque control amongst smokers or reduced tissue resistance, due to the constrictive effects of smoking on the gingival microcirculation. More recent evidence suggests that it is not smoking *per se* which is of aetiological importance but the underlying emotional state of the smoker whose habit reflects a certain personality type.

Mental or physical stress. It has been suggested that ANUG occurs in individuals subject to mental or physical stress whose gingival tissue, consequently, exhibits reduced resistance to disease. This might help to explain the apparent 'outbreaks' of ANUG. Since the condition is not contagious, outbreaks are more likely to be due to groups living or working in similar stressful situations. Such a theory would help to explain the widespread ANUG in the First World War ('trench mouth') and amongst groups of recruits in the modern army.

Impaired host resistance. When host resistance is impaired, the likelihood of severe gingival and periodontal disease is increased. Occasionally, gingival ulceration with a fibrinous pseudomembrane may be the earliest sign of acute leukaemia and, for this reason, any patient who does not respond as well as expected to local or systemic treatment should undergo haematological investigation. The management of oral lesions in acute leukaemia is complex and the reader is referred to the comprehensive review by Ferguson *et al.* (1978).

Recently, a high incidence of ANUG has been reported among victims of acquired immune deficiency syndrome (AIDS) and also in individuals with antibodies to human immunodeficiency virus (HIV) who have not developed AIDS.

Treatment

The treatment of ANUG varies with the severity of the condition. In all cases, local treatment of the condition is essential and, at least in the more severe cases, systemic treatment is also indicated. It may be argued that, because of the destructive nature of the ulcers and the safety of metronidazole, treatment with this drug should not be withheld.

Local treatment. The object of local treatment is a thorough débridement of the affected area over a period of a few visits, at each visit carrying out as much treatment as the discomfort felt by the patient will allow.

In severe cases it may only be possible to remove loose debris with cotton wool pellets soaked in hydrogen peroxide. The hydrogen peroxide is probably effective in two ways: the effervescence of the solution physically cleanses the area and the nascent oxygen released by the solution may be effective against anaerobic bacteria.

For the initial stages of débridement, an ultrasonic scaler is often of value. Ultrasonic scalers can be used with a minimum of discomfort and the spray produced by the scaler physically cleanses the area.

Gradually, the area should be cleaned more thoroughly until, eventually, a fine scale and polish has been carried out. Since the symptoms will have resolved before this stage is reached, there is a risk that treatment may be discontinued by the patient before then. The fact that tissue destruction may progress after the pain has been relieved needs to be carefully explained to the patient and the importance of completing a fine scale stressed.

Tooth extraction is contraindicated during ANUG and, if possible, should be delayed until the signs and symptoms have resolved.

Oral hygiene instruction. At each visit, the patient should also be given oral hygiene advice related to the condition. Depending on the severity of the pain, it may be necessary to recommend a soft toothbrush, but, in such cases, the patient should revert to a medium-textured brush as soon as the discomfort allows. Interdental cleaning is essential to achieve a good result and should be commenced as soon as discomfort allows.

Mouthwashes. An oxidising mouthwash such as sodium perborate (Bocasan) may be helpful in dislodging the slough and may have a direct antibacterial effect on the anaerobic bacteria which inhabit the ulcer. Prolonged use should be avoided because of the risk of borate poisoning.

Chlorhexidine, a broad-spectrum antiseptic and very effective in the prevention of dental plaque formation, appears to offer no benefit in the treatment of ANUG probably because it fails to penetrate the pseudomembrane. On the other hand, chlorhexidine may be valuable when mechanical plaque control is difficult following an episode of ANUG where soft-tissue interdental craters have formed.

Systemic treatment. If adequate débridement is carried out, systemic treatment should be unnecessary. However, because of the destructive nature of the disease, rapid resolution is desirable and there would seem to be little point in withholding systemic antibacterial therapy.

Metronidazole is the drug of choice and is usually administered in 200-mg doses, three times daily for three days. It should not be prescribed for patients who cannot or will not abstain from alcohol, since it will interact with alcohol to invoke headaches, nausea and vomiting and may even produce cardiac arrythmias, hypotension and collapse. Metronidazole, furthermore, potentiates coumarin anticoagulants.

Penicillin is at least as effective as metronidazole but produces more side-effects: hypersensitivity reactions and the selection of resistant organisms. It may, occasionally, be preferred to metronidazole; for example, if antibiotic prophylaxis is required to prevent infective endocarditis in a susceptible patient undergoing scaling for ANUG.

The use of drugs in the treatment of ANUG, to the exclusion of simultaneous local débridement, is to be deplored since it leads, in many cases, to recurrent episodes of the disease with periods of remission (during drug therapy) which are so short as to create a false impression of a chronic condition.

Follow-up care. The treatment of ANUG is not complete until a gingival architecture has been established which will allow adequate home care. Once the ulcers have healed, careful evaluation of the periodontal tissues should establish the likelihood of achieving a normal gingival architecture. Where soft-tissue craters are comparatively shallow and interdental oral hygiene is not seriously compromised, the chances of papillary regeneration are excellent. This process, however, may take many months and, since it will be inhibited by interdental plaque, close patient supervision is necessary.

Deeper soft-tissue craters will be found at sites where deep pockets existed previously, i.e. in cases of hyperplastic gingivitis or chronic periodontitis upon which ANUG has become superimposed. In these circumstances, little improvement in gingival contour may be anticipated without surgical intervention. A gingivectomy or flap procedure should be chosen in accordance with the principles expressed in Chapter 10, with the objective of achieving a physiological gingival sulcus and a gingival contour which will facilitate home care.

ACUTE HERPETIC STOMATITIS

Acute herpetic stomatitis or, as it is sometimes called, acute herpetic gingivostomatitis, is a systemic infection with the herpes simplex virus (Type 1) which is manifest by widespread intraoral vesicles and ulceration. It is not a form of plaque-associated periodontal disease but is considered here because the lesions may affect the gingiva predominantly and cause diagnostic confusion with ANUG.

Aetiology

Acute herpetic stomatitis is essentially a disease of early childhood, when the symptoms are usually mild and are probably often dismissed as 'teething'. However, as a result of improved living conditions, there is a reduced incidence in childhood and an increasing number of cases are diagnosed in adulthood, when the symptoms tend to be more severe. The virus is transmitted by contact with infected saliva. Virtually all adults have antibodies to this virus, indicating that they have suffered a primary infection at some time, albeit a mild one.

Clinical Presentation

In a severe case, the onset is sudden, with high fever, cervical lymphadenopathy and pain in the mouth and throat. The gingiva may become acutely inflamed, oedematous, and tender. Intra-epithelial vesicles form within 24 hours, usually on the tongue, buccal mucosa, palate and gingivae. The vesicles rupture early, giving numerous small round or irregular superficial ulcers which may coalesce. The ulcers have a greyish-yellow base and a distinct red halo. Sometimes the gingiva may remain red and painful without evidence of ulceration. Pain may interfere with eating and drinking and on occasions the patient may be reluctant to swallow.

A number of features of acute herpetic stomatitis distinguish it from ANUG. Systemic symptoms are more common and more severe; ulcers may affect not only the marginal gingiva, but also the attached gingiva and other parts of the oral mucosa; the gingival lesions are not necrotic. Unlike ANUG, acute herpetic stomatitis is a self-limiting condition which resolves in one or two weeks. The ulcers heal without residual deformity.

About 30% of individuals suffer recurrent infections later in life. These usually take the form of 'cold sores' on the lips (herpes labialis) but may present intraorally as a cluster of small, shallow ulcers with red irregular margins. In these cases there is usually no significant systemic upset.

Diagnosis

Usually the diagnosis can be made on clinical grounds alone. Laboratory tests may be helpful; the existence of a viral infection may be confirmed by cytological examination of a smear when typical viral damage may be noted; herpetic infection may be positively diagnosed by examining direct smears stained with specific fluorescent antisera, by viral isolation from tissue culture or, retrospectively, by serology.

Treatment

Treatment is supportive and includes a soft diet with adequate fluid intake. Bed rest and analgesics may also be necessary. Oral ulceration is managed with chlorhexidine mouthwash which will reduce secondary bacterial infection and maintain dental plaque control.

THE PERIODONTAL ABSCESS

In this chapter, the term 'periodontal abscess' refers to an infection where the gingival sulcus or periodontal pocket is the point of entry of the causative organisms. The term 'dental abscess' is reserved for an infection of pulpal origin.

The periodontal abscess is an acute suppurative inflammation due to bacteria from the sulcus or pocket establishing a nidus within the gingival or deeper periodontal tissues. A wide variety of organisms, facultative anaerobes and strict anaerobes, may be implicated in a pure or mixed infection. *Bacteroides* spp., *Eikenella corrodens* and anaerobic streptococci are common isolates. Since bacterial access to the periodontal connective tissues is a prerequisite for the development of such a lesion, periodontal abscesses are, not surprisingly, usually associated with a pre-existing subgingival plaque flora and traumatic penetration of pocket epithelium.

Trauma may be caused by toothbrush bristles, food impaction (e.g. fish bone) and dental procedures including scaling. Orthodontic therapy may also cause a periodontal abscess if a plaque-infected root surface is pressed against a pocket wall. Occlusal forces may also cause compression of the pocket wall.

Successful invasion of the periodontal tissue will be facilitated by failure of defence mechanisms and patients with uncontrolled diabetes, for example, will be predisposed to abscess formation.

Diagnosis

The periodontal abscess has a sudden onset. Pain will be present on biting and on percussion and may be continuous. There is usually swelling and tenderness of the overlying gingiva. Periodontal abscesses usually drain along the root surface to the pocket orifice although, in the case of deep pockets, they may drain through the alveolar process to produce a sinus opening in the attached gingiva. Because drainage usually occurs readily, the infection tends to remain localised. Extraoral swelling is uncommon.

The periodontal abscess possesses no special radiographic features, although it is commonly associated with a deep pocket and, therefore, with advanced marginal bone loss. 'Horizontal' or 'angular' bone loss may be evident.

The periodontal abscess must be differentiated from an abscess of pulpal origin. The dental abscess is associated with a non-vital pulp and usually presents as a periapical radiolucent lesion. Drainage tends to occur through alveolar mucosa rather than attached gingiva or the gingival sulcus. Dental abscesses may also occur on the lateral aspect of the root or in the furcation region if associated with lateral or accessory canals. This may lead to considerable diagnostic difficulty, especially if such an abscess should drain through the gingival sulcus (*see* Chapter 12).

Treatment

The prospects of achieving a return to periodontal health should first be assessed. The prognosis is poor if bone destruction is well advanced and there is a history of recurrent abscess formation. These teeth are best extracted. Extraction may be carried out immediately if the abscess is localised to a small area of periodontium, but otherwise may have to be postponed until the acute infection has been resolved.

Drainage can usually be encouraged by dilating the pocket with a periodontal probe or flat plastic instrument. Fluctuant gingival swellings, however, may require incision. A sample of pus should be obtained for culture and sensitivity tests. Gentle subgingival scaling should be carried out to remove calculus and foreign objects, if present, and the pocket irrigated with warm sterile saline. The patient should be advised to use hot saline mouthwashes at home, and these measures together will usually permit remission of the symptoms. Analgesics may be prescribed, if necessary. A systemic antibiotic should be prescribed for cellulitis or pyrexia. Penicillin is the drug of choice. Metronidazole may be a suitable alternative.

The patient should return two days later and local treatment, as described above, repeated. If at this visit, however, there has been no improvement in symptoms, an antibiotic should be prescribed according to the result of sensitivity tests. If an antibiotic was prescribed at the first visit and has been ineffective, it should be changed, again by reference to the sensitivity report.

As the symptoms resolve, oral hygiene instruction and superficial scaling should continue until sufficient time has elapsed for healing of the abscess site—about two months. Successful treatment is recognised by a considerable reduction in probing depth from an initial level. A pathological pocket, albeit with a reduced depth, may still exist and should be subjected to definitive treatment according to the principles expressed in Chapter 7. This may involve subgingival scaling and root planing or surgical intervention.

Sometimes the acute symptoms disappear but a chronic draining lesion remains. This may signify a continuing rapid, destructive process and may be a sign of bad prognosis. To arrest the destructive process in these cases, early surgical intervention is indicated following satisfactory completion of hygiene therapy and preparation of a definitive treatment plan.

Although the periodontal abscess is associated with rapid and extensive destruction of periodontal tissue and the occurrence of very deep pockets, it would appear that sufficient periodontal ligament cells may survive the acute destructive process to regenerate a connective tissue attachment once the acute lesion has resolved. The potential for regeneration, however, will no longer exist if the remnants of the old ligament are destroyed by enthusiastic instrumentation. Deep scaling, root planing and subgingival curettage of periodontal abscess sites during the acute phase is, therefore, quite inappropriate. Subgingival scaling should not extend beyond the apical extent of subgingival calculus, which is the best available guide to the level of pre-existing chronic disease.

Traditionally, systemic antibacterial drug therapy for abscesses of the oral tissues has been mainly reserved for severe infections. However, in the case of a periodontal abscess, there may be some justification for employing antibacterial drug therapy even for well-localised infections, since conventional mechanical therapy carries the risk of permanent destruction of periodontal attachment.

REFERENCES

Loesche W. J., Syed S. A., Laughton B. E., Stoll J. (1982). The bacteriology of acute necrotising ulcerative gingivitis. *Journal of Periodontology*; **53**: 223–30.

Ferguson M. M., Stephen K. W., Dagg J. H., Hunter I. P. (1978). The presentation and management of oral lesions in leukaemia. *Journal of Dentistry*; **6**: 201–6.

FURTHER READING

Falkler W. A., Jr., Martin S. A., Vincent J. W., Tall B. D. (1987). A clinical, demographic and microbiologic study of ANUG patients in an urban dental school. *Journal of Clinical Periodontology*; **14**: 307–14.

Johnson B. D., Engel D. (1986). Acute necrotizing ulcerative gingivitis—a review of diagnosis, etiology and treatment. *Journal of Periodontology*; **57**: 141–50.

Sabiston C. B., Jr. (1986). A review and proposal for the etiology of acute necrotizing gingivitis. *Journal of Clinical Periodontology*; **13**: 727–34.

Smith R. G., Davies R. M. (1986). Acute lateral periodontal abscesses. *British Dental Journal*; **161**: 176–8.

Chapter 19

Desquamative Gingivitis

'Desquamative gingivitis' (Fig. 19.1) refers to a painful gingival lesion or lesions characterised by a smooth, red, glistening surface with a tendency to desquamation and haemorrhage on slight trauma. It may affect both the free and attached gingiva. It is not a specific disease entity but rather a manifestation of many different conditions. The definition is usually extended to include vesiculobullous and ulcerative lesions.

AETIOLOGY

Unlike marginal periodontal disease, desquamative gingivitis is not caused by the accumulation of bacterial plaque on cervical tooth regions or its subgingival growth. Although both conditions may be present simultaneously, their coexistence is purely coincidental.

Formerly, desquamative gingivitis was related to the menopause and hormone therapy was often attempted. In the late 1950s, however, it was recognised to be a manifestation of

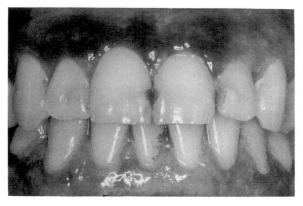

Fig. 19.1 *Desquamative gingivitis affecting the 3/ to /1 region. This was a manifestation of atrophic lichen planus. Note the contrast between maxillary and mandibular gingivae.*

several disease processes. Nowadays, the underlying disorder can be identified in the majority of cases, the commonest diagnoses being lichen planus and benign mucous membrane pemphigoid.

Lichen Planus

Lichen planus is a relatively common chronic disease of unknown aetiology which affects the skin and mucous membranes. Often, lesions are confined to the mouth. Oral lichen planus, which occurs predominantly in adult females, is characterised by white striations, papules and plaque-like lesions, primarily on buccal mucosa and lateral borders of the tongue. The lesions of lichen planus, as well as being keratotic, may be atrophic or erosive, particularly where they involve the gingiva, giving rise to the diagnosis of 'desquamative gingivitis'.

Gingival involvement is present in 10–20% of oral lesions. Diagnosis may be difficult if the lesions are confined to the gingiva, since the classical keratotic appearance is often absent. Nevertheless, a definitive diagnosis is important to exclude other, more serious diseases which may mimic lichen planus.

The diagnosis of lichen planus can often be established by biopsy studies. The microscopic appearance of gingival lesions is comparable to that of lichen planus involvement elsewhere in the mouth. White lesions will present orthokeratosis or parakeratosis, acanthosis, liquefaction degeneration of the basal epithelial layer and a dense subepithelial lymphocytic infiltrate. Atrophic or erosive lesions, on the other hand, show thinning of the epithelium or ulceration and often the picture is obscured by a non-specific inflammatory infiltrate.

Direct immunofluorescent studies of gingival biopsy material may reveal globular deposits in the lamina propria, and fibrin deposits along the basement membrane. These findings are suggestive but not diagnostic of lichen planus. Indirect immunofluorescence will be negative.

In contrast to other oral lesions of lichen planus, gingival lesions tend to be painful. Patients may complain of a burning sensation and of extreme discomfort on eating and toothbrushing. Reassurance should be given and chlorhexidine mouthwash prescribed if only to achieve some measure of plaque control and reduce the incidence of secondary infection. Periodic scaling, including subgingival scaling, may also be of benefit.

Topical steroid applications may be used in more severe cases. Fluorinated corticosteroid cream, applied two or three times daily, has been recommended recently (Nisengard and Rogers, 1987). If the lesion is painful but not extensive, excision may be worthwhile. Systemic steroids are rarely justified. The oral disease may last for several years although skin lesions rarely persist beyond 18 months.

Benign Mucous Membrane Pemphigoid

This is a chronic vesiculobullous disorder occurring most commonly in females, with a peak incidence in the fifth decade. The oral mucosa is almost invariably affected while other mucosae, particularly the conjuctivae, are sometimes involved. Skin lesions are much less common and tend to be adjacent to mucosal surfaces.

The most frequent site of oral involvement is the gingiva, which may appear red and glistening and produce vesicles or bullae. These are often blood-filled and persist for a day or two before rupturing to form erosions. Conjunctival lesions may heal with scarring and corneal adhesions are a serious complication of the disease.

Microscopically, subepithelial blister formation may be evident, with an underlying non-specific inflammatory infiltrate. These appearances are suggestive but not diagnostic, and depend on obtaining a biopsy specimen of an intact bulla. Perilesional or relatively normal tissue may, however, be examined by direct immunofluorescence to reveal immune deposits along the basement membrane, providing confirmation of the diagnosis. Indirect immunofluorescence is usually negative.

Lesions confined to the mouth should be treated by local measures if possible, as for lichen planus. In the case of pemphigoid, bullae will tend to form at sites of trauma. Toothbrushing must often, therefore, be restricted or modified and chlorhexidine mouthwash should be used as the principal plaque control agent. Systemic treatment with dapsone is usually reserved for ocular involvement. Dapsone is an anti-bacterial drug used primarily in the treatment of leprosy and dermatitis herpetiformis. Systemic steroid therapy is usually ineffective.

When benign mucous membrane pemphigoid is diagnosed, referral to an ophthalmologist should be considered.

Other Dermatological Diseases

Erythema multiforme, lupus erythematosus, bullous pemphigoid, psoriasis, pemphigus vulgaris and pemphigus vegetans are dermatological diseases which may occasionally manifest desquamative gingival lesions.

Adverse Drug Reactions

The oral mucosa is the seat of adverse reactions to a very large number of drugs. These reactions may take the form of vesicles, bullae, ulcers and erosions and the gingiva is sometimes affected.

The 'aspirin burn' is a well-recognised example of a drug having local irritant effects. Chlorhexidine mouthwash may also cause desquamative lesions in susceptible individuals. It has been suggested that this is due to precipitation of the protective mucin layer by chlorhexidine, and is related to the concentration of the drug.

Desquamative gingival lesions may result from contact hypersensitivity to toothpaste, mouthwashes, cosmetics, chewing gums, iodine, essential oils and many other substances.

A variety of drug eruptions may manifest themselves on the oral mucosa. Barbiturates, chlordiazepoxide and tetracyclines may cause a fixed drug eruption, a cell-mediated hypersensitivity reaction manifest as ulceration, bullae, erythema or superficial erosions. Lichenoid eruptions may occur, clinically and histologically similar to lichen planus lesions, in response to a wide range of drugs such as methyldopa, amiphenazole and phenothiazines.

Systemic anti-inflammatory agents suppress the regenerative capacity of oral mucosa. This effect is shared by cytotoxic drugs which also cause granulocytopenia, reducing mucosal resistance to infection.

DIFFERENTIAL DIAGNOSIS

A careful history is essential to identify any existing dermatological or systemic disease which may be the cause of the gingival lesions. An accurate drug history will help to identify a drug-induced disorder. The majority of patients with desquamative gingivitis who present without any relevant medical history are likely to be suffering from atrophic or erosive lichen planus or benign mucous membrane pemphigoid. Examination of skin and ocular lesions, if present, should be undertaken and gingival biopsy, using light microscopy, will usually be necessary to establish the diagnosis. Occasionally, immunofluorescent studies of perilesional gingival biopsy specimens or indirect immunofluorescent examination of serum for epithelial or basement membrane antibodies must be undertaken for confirmation.

The differential diagnosis of desquamative gingivitis is reviewed by Nisengard and Neiders (1981).

REFERENCES

Nisengard R. J., Neiders M. (1981). Desquamative lesions of the gingiva. *Journal of Periodontology*; **52**: 500–10.
Nisengard R. J., Rogers R. S. (1987). The treatment of desquamative gingival lesions. *Journal of Periodontology*; **58**: 167–72.

Chapter 20

Growing Points in Periodontal Research

In preceding chapters, we have sought to emphasise the effective diagnostic and therapeutic procedures *currently available*. The purpose of this final chapter is to present a synopsis of some aspects of clinical periodontal research, not yet wholly suitable for practical application but which continue to generate a substantial literature.

BACTERIOLOGICAL EVALUATION IN PERIODONTITIS

Studies on the Predominant Cultivable Flora

There are over 200 bacterial species associated with the gingival crevice and most of these organisms have been found in subgingival plaque. There is no convincing evidence to support the theory of a single periodontal pathogen. However, it is recognised that some subgingival bacteria will play a larger role than others. Those listed in Table 20.1 are common isolates, frequently constituting more than 2–3% and sometimes more than 50% of the cultivable subgingival flora, and possessing various virulence factors. All are members of the normal oral flora and are found, albeit in much smaller proportions, in healthy sites.

As microbiological techniques improve it seems certain that other organisms will be added to the list of candidate pathogens. At present, it is still not possible to culture or identify all plaque bacteria or to grow them in the same proportions as present in the sample: sensitive organisms may be lost in the transport medium and there is no suitable culture medium which will support the most fastidious organisms. Spirochaetes, for example, are easily recognisable by direct microscopy of plaque samples and often account for more than 50% of organisms present. However, they comprise many different species and are very difficult to cultivate. The bacteriological picture is further obscured by the

Table 20.1. *Common isolates from subgingival plaque (in alphabetical order)*

Bacterium	Characteristics		
Bacteroides gingivalis	Gram −ve	non-motile	anaerobic rod
Bacteroides intermedius	Gram −ve	non-motile	anaerobic rod
Capnocytophaga species	Gram −ve	motile	capnophilic* rod
Eikenella corrodens	Gram −ve	non-motile	facultative rod
Eubacterium species	Gram +ve	non-motile	anaerobic rod
Fusobacterium nucleatum	Gram −ve	non-motile	anaerobic rod
Actinobacillus actinomycetemcomitans	Gram −ve	non-motile	capnophilic* rod
Treponema species	Gram −ve	motile	anaerobic spirochaete
Wolinella recta	Gram −ve	motile	anaerobic curved rod

* Capnophilic = CO_2 dependent.

recent recognition that most of the organisms listed in Table 20.1, including *A. actinomycetemcomitans* and both species of *Bacteroides* exhibit heterogeneity, some strains being more virulent than others.

Efforts have been made to link different forms of periodontitis with different bacterial species. This concept of *bacterial specificity* considers periodontal disease to be a group of specific infections each associated with different and specific groups of micro-organisms. For instance, the high proportional recovery of *A. actinomycetemcomitans* from many juvenile periodontitis patients is thought to support the bacterial specificity theory. However, attempts to label other clinical disease entities with a specific microflora have met with little success. The different forms of periodontitis (Appendix III) are clinically very ill-defined and there appears to be considerable overlap in bacteriological findings between them. Furthermore, within the same mouth, different sites with similar clinical characteristics have been shown often to harbour different organisms.

Association of Certain Organisms with Phases of Destruction

Periodontitis is known to behave in a variety of different ways. Lesions may persist in a quiescent form, may progress slowly, possibly with short periods of destruction and inactivity, or may exhibit acute bursts of activity. It seems reasonable to propose that these different forms of behaviour may reflect the composition of subgingival plaque. This supposition has been investigated both by direct examination of pocket samples using dark-field or phase-contrast microscopy and by cultural studies.

Microscopic analysis of plaque samples has shown that 'healthy' gingival sites are dominated by coccoid cells while 'diseased' sites contain increased proportions of motile rods and spirochaetes. Spirochaetes alone may account for more than 50% of the organisms present in a 'diseased' site and generally greater proportions are present in deep pockets than in shallow pockets. However, not all patients or sites with advanced periodontitis have high counts of motile rods and spirochaetes.

When periodontitis is treated by mechanical débridement or antibacterial drug therapy, the percentage of motile rods and spirochaetes diminishes, but failure to establish and maintain a physiological gingival sulcus leads to a gradual return to pretreatment levels.

A number of studies have considered the possibility that motile rods or spirochaetes might be indicator organisms of a pathogenic microflora and of impending tissue destruction. However, great variability in the percentages of these organisms has been observed between sites, whether active or inactive, in the same patient. Only by examining bacterial samples pooled from the deepest pocket in each sextant has it been possible to demonstrate a positive correlation between the proportions of subgingival spirochaetes and motile rods and susceptibility of human subjects to periodontal deterioration (Listgarten and Levin, 1981).

As an alternative to expensive and time-consuming cultural methods, it was perhaps inevitable that dark-field and phase-contrast microscopy would be explored early as a possible chairside facility in clinical periodontal practice. Direct microscopy has proven too unreliable, however, and since it cannot differentiate between the many species of suspected pathogens, it seems unlikely to merit further consideration.

Cultural studies have focused on the *non*-motile *B. gingivalis*, *B. intermedius* and *A. actinomycetemcomitans* and there is some evidence to suggest that a high proportional recovery of any one of these organisms may reflect the existence of progressive periodontitis. This finding is based on a number of investigations, reviewed by Slots (1986), in which these organisms singly or in combination were highly prevalent in sites of progressive periodontitis. It was further suggested (Bragd *et al.* 1987) that critical recovery levels of 0·01% for *A. actinomycetemcomitans*, 0·1% for *B. gingivalis* and 2·5% for *B. intermedius* could be used to distinguish non-progressing from progressing periodontal sites with reasonable confidence. It must be understood, however, that bacteriological sampling in this study was carried out *after* destruction had taken place and it is possible that the organisms identified may simply be those normally found in *deeper* pockets, representing the aftermath of a changed environment rather than causative agents. Indeed, longitudinal studies to determine which species are present or increased during destruction as compared with inactive sites of *similar depth* in the same subjects suggest that activity is associated with different bacterial species in different patients. No one species has been shown to be present in all cases of any clinical category of periodontitis.

A major weakness of investigations which seek to identify the organisms associated with phases of periodontal destruction is the absence of any method, clinical or laboratory, which can record the destructive episode *as it occurs*. Radiographic changes of crestal bone level and clinical measurements of loss of attachment will, at best, identify *recent* destructive activity. The chances of taking a bacterial sample from the right place at the right time to represent actively progressing disease are small.

Bacterial Invasion

Traditionally, periodontitis has been regarded as an infectious process where the aetiological agents lie *within* the pocket, their metabolic products diffusing into the soft tissues to produce an inflammatory response. In the last decade, however, there have been many reports of apparent bacterial invasion of the pocket soft tissues, even to the level of the alveolar bone crest. Nisengard and Bascones (1987) have compiled recent evidence which supports the concept of bacterial invasion. 'Invading' organisms are typically Gram-negative rods or spirochaetes. Using immunocytochemistry techniques, *A. actinomycetemcomitans* and *Treponema vincenti* have been identified within connective tissue of the pocket wall in periodontitis. Clearly, any bacteria capable of overcoming host defences and invading the tissues are of special aetiological importance, and it has been suggested that invading organisms may be responsible for the destructive phases of periodontitis.

While the *presence* of organisms within biopsy specimens is not in dispute, many investigators argue that the bacteria are probably passively introduced either during occlusal function (if the tooth is loose) or surgically implanted inadvertently when the biopsy is taken.

Implications for Clinical Practice

Microbiological tests in clinical periodontal practice have been advocated: to determine the causative agent; to determine sites of active tissue destruction; to assist in treatment planning for new and 'refractory' patients; to monitor the effects of treatment and to decide on a recall interval (Genco *et al.*, 1986). However, reliance on bacteriological data can only be justified when most of the causative bacteria are known and can be readily detected, and it is clear from the growing literature on the subject that this is not the case. At the present time, it would be quite wrong to withhold treatment from a patient whose pockets did not yield any of the currently recognised pathogens on culture. Even if the pocket inhabitants were indeed 'harmless' organisms at the time of sampling, the very existence of a subgingival flora must be considered a long-term threat because of the possibility of overgrowth of more virulent types in the future. It is difficult, therefore, to see how present knowledge of the microbiology of periodontitis should alter traditional therapeutic approaches, except, perhaps, when dealing with juvenile periodontitis.

Sampling for *A. actinomycetemcomitans* in juvenile periodontitis is probably the only bacteriological test which may contribute to the treatment of periodontitis at the present time. The high virulence of this organism and its reported ability to invade the pocket connective tissues may be sufficient grounds for tetracycline therapy as an adjunct to root instrumentation in some cases (*see* Chapter 15).

The concept of identifying and subsequently eliminating a specific pathogen by chemotherapeutic means may be an attractive one. However, since the potential periodontal pathogens are indigenous bacteria, it is neither possible nor desirable to eradicate them. At the moment, the only way to achieve a permanent reduction of the most virulent species is to maintain a plaque ecology unfavourable for these species: by removing subgingival plaque and keeping supragingival plaque and gingivitis at a minimum. This is the basis for conventional, mechanical treatment of periodontitis.

ANTIBACTERIAL CHEMOTHERAPY

Although this topic has a vast literature, the purpose of the present discussion is merely to explore some of the more contentious issues.

Pocket Irrigation with Chlorhexidine

Chlorhexidine, although safe and effective as an inhibitor of supragingival plaque, does not, when used as a mouthwash, enter periodontal pockets and is, therefore, ineffective in the treatment of periodontitis.

Pockets, however, can be irrigated with chlorhexidine using a blunt needle inserted 3 mm within the pocket and numerous studies (reviewed by Wennström *et al.*, 1987) have been carried out to test the efficacy of chlorhexidine irrigation as an adjunct to root instrumentation in the treatment of periodontitis. Generally, results have been disappointing since no effect on attachment levels has been demonstrated, although in one series of studies, reduced gingival bleeding and probing depths were obtained by the adjunctive effect of *daily* chlorhexidine irrigation. The subjects in those studies, however, did not carry out interdental cleaning, and the reduction in gingivitis which was achieved could be explained by the effect of the irrigant on approximal supragingival plaque formation at the sites of needle insertion. It seems, therefore, that pocket irrigation with chlorhexidine has little to commend it other than for its mechanical flushing effect.

Chlorhexidine's failure to have a significant effect on the subgingival microflora may be partly attributed to its inability to influence preformed plaque and partly to the lack of time for adsorption of the chlorhexidine to the subgingival root surface and soft-tissue pocket wall. Thus an effective concentration of the agent within the pocket would not be established and maintained. The need to maintain optimal concentrations of antimicrobial agents for use in periodontal pockets has led to the testing of various slow-release devices.

Slow-release Devices

To be clinically acceptable, such devices must be easy to insert and retain *in situ* and less time consuming and uncomfortable than conventional periodontal treatment. So far, these problems have not been adequately resolved, although many different methods of controlled local drug delivery have been tested, demonstrating clinical effects comparable to conventional instrumentation. These include the use of hollow cellulose acetate fibres, cellulose-based dialysis tubing and acrylic resin strips, filled or impregnated with chlorhexidine, tetracycline or metronidazole.

This line of research has led to the investigation of tetracycline-containing monolithic fibres of ethylene vinyl acetate (Goodson *et al.*, 1985). These have been shown to maintain a concentration of at least 50 μg/ml in the periodontal pocket for a period of 10 days. This should be compared with a concentration in gingival fluid of 5–14 μg/ml sustained for 3 hours, achievable by systemic administration of a 250-mg dose of tetracycline.

Because all mechanical devices tend to be pushed out of the pocket by gingival fluid, research has extended to biodegradable adhesives but their value has not yet been fully assessed.

Systemic Antibacterial Agents in the Treatment of Periodontitis

In recent years, treatment strategies involving systemic chemo-therapy have been tested in the management of chronic periodontitis. The drugs which have proved most successful in clinical trials are metronidazole and tetracycline, to which many of the putative periodontal pathogens are sensitive.

Metronidazole is excreted in gingival fluid in concentrations equal to those in serum. Strict anaerobes such as *B. gingivalis* and *B. intermedius* are sensitive and the development of resistant organisms has not been observed. However, most facultative anaerobes and capnophilic organisms such as *A. actinomy-cetemcomitans* are inherently resistant to this antibacterial agent. Tetracycline accumulates in the pocket in concentrations which are higher than those in serum. It is a broad-spectrum bacteriostatic antibiotic, effective against the majority of periodontal pathogens and notably against *A. actinomycetem-comitans* and *Capnocytophaga*. Toxic side-effects are minimal. However, the emergence of resistant organisms is a problem wherever tetracycline is used.

Many studies have been carried out to assess the effect on periodontitis of systemic antimicrobial therapy with or without mechanical débridement. Nevertheless, it is impossible to draw any firm conclusions since many of these studies either involved small numbers of subjects, lacked parallel control groups or were of short duration.

Generally, both metronidazole and tetracycline, used without mechanical débridement, were inferior to scaling and root planing alone. This is not surprising when the modes of action of these drugs are considered: metronidazole, although bactericidal against strict anaerobes, will leave unaffected the facultative and capnophilic segment of the pocket flora to which many important pathogens belong; tetracycline, although active against most of the periodontal pathogens, is bacteriostatic and will achieve only temporary suppression of these organisms.

Minor benefits have been observed by some investigators when metronidazole has been used as an adjunct to mechanical débridement. However, further studies are needed if indications are to be established for the use of metronidazole in the treatment of periodontitis. Metronidazole is an important drug in the treatment of surgical and gynaecological sepsis involving colonic anaerobes, and its indiscriminate use in the treatment of chronic periodontitis cannot be condoned lest its role in medicine and surgery be compromised. As for adjunctive tetracycline, there is some evidence to support its use in the treatment of those forms of periodontitis where *A. actinomycetemcomitans* has been isolated. This organism may be capable of invading the pocket soft tissues, thereby surviving non-surgical scaling procedures. It has been linked with juvenile periodontitis and conditions for tetracycline therapy are outlined in Chapter 14.

NEW ATTACHMENT THERAPY

The ultimate aim of periodontal therapy must be the regeneration of predisease quantities of healthy supporting tissue comprising new alveolar bone, periodontal ligament and cementum. At present, we are obliged to accept as a realistic aim, the restoration to health of remaining periodontal support, i.e. the arrest but not reversal of connective tissue attachment loss. During healing, epithelial reattachment to the previously diseased root surface occurs, but it seems likely that any areas of apparently 'new' connective tissue attachment are of healthy connective tissue attachment disrupted for the first time by surgery. Substantial research work suggests that wound healing with the formation of a new connective tissue attachment would be a process of great complexity. The critical factors in this process are summarised below.

Bone Grafts

Early attempts at regenerative surgery involved various types of bone graft, packed into angular bone defects and covered with soft tissue. Materials tested include fresh and frozen iliac crest autogenous cancellous bone and marrow, frozen allogenic iliac cancellous bone and marrow, and freeze-dried allogenic cortical bone. More recently, inert ceramic grafts comprising biodegradable tricalcium phosphate and non-resorbable hydroxyapatite have been used. There is no evidence that any of these grafts facilitates connective tissue attachment to the root surface, epithelialisation of the root-surface–graft-tissue interface occurring instead. Indeed, the grafts even appear to have limited osteogenic potential, several studies having observed little or no advantage to osseous grafting over non-grafted controls with respect to the amount of bone-fill achieved.

Root Surface Conditioning

Citric acid has been shown to dissolve the smear layer formed by root planing, to detoxify remaining root surface contaminant, and to demineralise the dentine surface, exposing collagen fibrils of the dentine matrix. These exposed fibrils are thought to improve the adhesion, proliferation and migration of fibroblasts on the root surface and to interdigitate with newly formed collagen fibrils in the healing tissue. Thus, citric acid conditioning may facilitate early adhesion of the fibrin coagulum to the root surface, thereby preventing apical migration of epithelial cells, as well as setting in motion the desired maturation and organisation of granulation tissue. The effect of citric acid has been tested in experimental animals with conflicting results and in humans generally with very little success.

Surgical Technique

A traditional reverse-bevel incision, rather than an intracrevicular incision, must be used so that when the flap is readapted to the root surface it will be virtually devoid of epithelium on its inner surface. Furthermore, a technique should be employed which will leave the root-surface–coagulum interface protected from mechanical injury during healing. Failure to accomplish this postoperative flap stability may encourage epithelial colonisation of the root surface. The difficulties in obtaining adequate wound protection may explain why success with citric acid root conditioning is frequently not achieved.

Root Resorption

In new attachment studies in animals, citric acid root conditioning has proved to be a two-edged sword. Although achieving a measure of new connective tissue attachment by preventing epithelial down-growth, it exposes the root surface to the activity of resorbing giant cells originating from gingival connective tissue and alveolar bone. Generally, the incidence and extent of root resorption increases with increase in the surface area of initial connective tissue attachment obtained. It remains possible that this phenomenon of root resorption is confined to the animal models used. Root resorption is an infrequent and late complication of human studies. However, new attachment formation following regenerative surgery in humans is also an infrequent occurrence.

Periodontal Ligament Progenitor Cells

As healing proceeds, it will be necessary for the root surface to be populated by periodontal ligament cells from adjacent intact periodontium and studies are already in progress to investigate chemotactic mechanisms which could accelerate the migration of these progenitor cells. It has been shown that only cells originating from the periodontal ligament are capable of producing a connective tissue attachment without the risk of root resorption. This has been achieved in animals and humans by a process known as guided tissue regeneration. This involves the placement of a porous teflon membrane (Gore-tex®) underneath the surgical flap, extending from the *outer* surface of the reduced alveolar process to the crown of the tooth above the gingival margin. Thus, both the epithelial and connective tissue components of the gingiva can be excluded from the root surface, allowing it to become populated exclusively by periodontal ligament cells. Follow-up surgery is necessary to remove the membrane. With this technique, root resorption has not been observed, at least in the short term. This is an entirely different approach to the problem from that exemplified by citric acid root conditioning, but many practical difficulties need to be overcome before guided tissue regeneration can make a significant contribution to periodontal therapy.

REFERENCES

Bacterial Evaluation in Periodontitis

Bragd L., Dahlen G., Wikstrom M., Slots J. (1987). The capability of *Actinobacillus actinomycetemcomitans*, *Bacteroides gingivalis* and *Bacteroides intermedius* to indicate progressive periodontitis; a retrospective study. *Journal of Clinical Periodontology*; **14**: 95–9.

Genco R. J., Zambon J. J., Christersson L. A. (1986). Use and interpretation of microbiological assays in periodontal diseases. *Oral Microbiology and Immunology*; **1**: 73–9.

Listgarten M. A., Levin S. (1981). Positive correlation between the proportions of subgingival spirochetes and motile bacteria and susceptibility of human subjects to periodontal deterioration. *Journal of Clinical Periodontology*; **8**: 122–38.

Nisengard R., Bascones A. (1987). Bacterial invasion in periodontal disease: a workshop. *Journal of Periodontology*; **58**: 331–9.

Slots J. (1986). Bacterial specificity in adult periodontitis. A summary of recent work. *Journal of Clinical Periodontology*; **13**: 912–17.

Antibacterial Chemotherapy

Goodson J. M., Offenbacher S., Farr D. H., Hogan P. E. (1985). Periodontal disease treatment by local drug delivery. *Journal of Periodontology*; **56**: 265–73.

Wennström J. L., Heijl L., Dahlen G., Grondahl K. (1987). Periodic subgingival antimicrobial irrigation of periodontal pockets (1).

Clinical observations. *Journal of Clinical Periodontology*; **14**: 541–50.

FURTHER READING

Bacterial Evaluation in Periodontitis

Greenstein G., Polson A. (1985). Microscopic monitoring of pathogens associated with periodontal disease—a review. *Journal of Periodontology*; **56**: 740–7.

Liakoni H., Barber P., Newman H. N. (1987). Bacterial penetration of pocket soft tissues in chronic adult and juvenile periodontitis cases. An ultrastructural study. *Journal of Clinical Periodontology*; **14**: 22–8.

Slots J., Listgarten M. (1988). *Bacteroides gingivalis, Bacteroides intermedius* and *Actinobacillus actinomycetemcomitans* in human periodontal diseases. *Journal of Clinical Periodontology*; **15**: 85–93.

Socransky S. S., Haffajee A. D., Smith G. L. F., Dzink J. L. (1987). Difficulties encountered in the search for etiologic agents of destructive periodontal diseases. *Journal of Clinical Periodontology*; **14**: 588–93.

Theilade E. (1986). The non-specific theory in microbial etiology of inflammatory periodontal diseases. *Journal of Clinical Periodontology*; **13**: 905–11.

Antibacterial Chemotherapy

Addy M. (1986). Chlorhexidine compared with other locally delivered antimicrobials. A short review. *Journal of Clinical Periodontology*; **13**: 957–64.

F. D. I. Technical Report No. 26 (1987) Topical and systemic antimicrobial agents in the treatment of chronic gingivitis and periodontitis. *International Dental Journal*; **37**: 52–62.

Gjermo P. (1986). Chemotherapy in juvenile periodontitis. *Journal of Clinical Periodontology*; **13**: 982–6.

Greenstein G. (1987). Effects of subgingival irrigation on periodontal status. *Journal of Periodontology*; **58**: 827–36.

Heijl L. (1985). The use of chemotherapy in the management of subgingival microbiota. In *The Dental Annual* . (Derrick D. D., ed.) pp. 58–72. Bristol: John Wright.

Newman H. N. (1986). Modes of application of anti-plaque chemicals. *Journal of Clinical Periodontology*; **13**: 965–74.

Van Palenstein Helderman W. H. (1986). Is antibiotic therapy justified in the treatment of human chronic inflammatory periodontal disease? *Journal of Clinical Periodontology*; **13**: 932–8.

New Attachment Therapy

Egelberg J. (1987). Regeneration and repair of periodontal tissues. *Journal of Periodontal Research*; **22**: 233–42.

Nyman S., Gottlow J., Lindhe J., Karring T., Wennström J. (1987). New attachment formation by guided tissue regeneration. *Journal of Periodontal Research*; **22**: 252–4.

Polson A. M. (1986). The root surface and regeneration; present therapeutic limitations and future biologic potentials. *Journal of Clinical Periodontology*; **13**: 995–9.

Examination and Treatment Planning Chart

EXPLANATORY NOTES

Numerous methods exist for recording clinical periodontal data. The chart illustrated combines the advantages of a pictorial system for rapid identification of particular teeth with space for numerical data. All the clinical data may be recorded on this type of chart and space is provided to record the treatment requirements of individual teeth. This system of charting, furthermore, places an emphasis on precise identification of diseased sites.

The chart may be used at the patient's first visit or at any subsequent visit, either during treatment or at recall. Use of this chart is particularly advised following completion of hygiene therapy, except for the simplest and most straightforward cases.

Data are collected by making separate circuits of the mouth for each pathological feature. This is less time consuming than collecting all the different types of data for each tooth in turn. The following examination and treatment planning procedure is recommended.

a) *Missing teeth*
   Missing teeth are recorded by deleting the relevant portions of the charted dentition.

b) *Pocket depths*
   Six aspects of every tooth are probed: distolingual, mid-lingual, mesiolingual, distobuccal, mid-buccal and mesiobuccal. This is carried out by examining an entire arch, first the lingual surfaces, probing three aspects of each tooth, and then repeating the procedure for buccal surfaces. The depth of every pathological (inflamed or bleeding) pocket, whether a contained gingival lesion or a perio-dontitis lesion, is noted. Healthy sites should not be scored.

c) *Mobility scores*
   The mobility of each tooth is measured and scores are

EXAMINATION AND TREATMENT PLAN CHART

Upper arch treatment plan	Furcations	Mobility	Pockets		Furcations	Mobility	Pockets	Lower arch treatment plan

recorded using a numerical system such as the Miller index, as follows:

> Grade 1—slight mobility
> Grade 2—moderate mobility up to 1 mm in a horizontal direction
> Grade 3—mobility greater than 1 mm in a horizontal direction, rotation or depression

d) *Furcation lesions*

> Grade 1—up to 3 mm horizontal attachment loss
> Grade 2—over 3 mm horizontal attachment loss but not 'through-and-through'
> Grade 3—a 'through-and-through' lesion

The furcation score is marked on the chart according to the site of the lesion, i.e. buccal, lingual, mesial or distal.

e) *Other clinical findings*

According to the needs of the clinician, additional information may be obtained and recorded: caries and overhanging restorations may be marked on the relevant tooth in red and black ink, respectively; unerupted teeth may be circled in black; non-vital teeth may be circled in red; plaque, gingivitis and recession scores may be recorded by adding vertical columns alongside the furcation column, etc.

f) *The treatment plan*

The treatment needs of individual teeth are recorded. With regard to periodontal therapy, the dentition should be divided into segments, sextants, quadrants or any other convenient grouping. A treatment sequence may then be drawn up on a separate sheet of paper to include all aspects of dental and periodontal therapy.

Periodontal Screening System for General Dental Practice

(Reprinted with kind permission of the British Society of Periodontology.)

The system described below originated in the document 'PERIODONTOLOGY IN GENERAL DENTAL PRACTICE IN THE UNITED KINGDOM – A FIRST POLICY STATEMENT' to which the reader is refered and from which this document is extracted. It is available on application to the Secretary, The British Society of Periodontology.

For examination the dentition is divided into sextants as shown:

UPPER

RIGHT	17-14	13-23	24-27	LEFT
	47-44	43-33	34-37	

LOWER

The use of a periodontal probe is mandatory. The recommended probe has a ball end 0·5 mm diameter. A colour-coded area extends from 3·5 to 5·5 mm. Probing force should not exceed 20–25 gm.

The probe tip is gently inserted into the gingival pocket and the depth of insertion read against the colour coding. The total extent of the pocket should be explored, conveniently by 'walking' the probe around the pocket. At least six points on each tooth should be examined: mesio buccal, mid buccal, distobuccal and the corresponding lingual sites.

For each sextant only the highest score or* is recorded. A sextant with only one tooth is recorded as missing and the tooth score included in the adjacent sextant. A simple box chart is used to record the scores for each sextant (see Fig.1).

FIG 1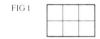

Code 4:
Coloured area of probe disappears into the pocket indicating probing depth of at least 6 mm.

Code 3:
Coloured area of probe remains **partly** visible in the deepest pocket in the sextant.

Code 2:
Coloured area of probe remains **completely** visible in the deepest pocket in the sextant. Supra or subgingival calculus is detected or the defective margin of a filling or crown.

Code 1:
Coloured area of probe remains **completely** visible in the deepest pocket in the sextant. No calculus or defective margins are detected. There is bleeding after gentle probing.

Code 0:
Healthy gingival tissues with no bleeding after gentle probing.

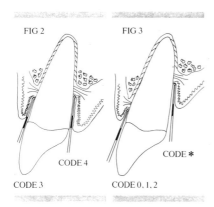

FIG 2   FIG 3

CODE 4

CODE 3

CODE *

CODE 0, 1, 2

In addition to these scores we recommend that the symbol * should be **substituted** for the sextant score whenever a furcation involvement is noted or there is total attachment loss of 7 mm or more at any site within that sextant.

*Code *:*
Denotes two special features causing periodontal problems, namely:
Furcation involvement.
Recession **plus** probing depth totals 7 mm or more.

Whenever Codes 4 or * are recorded the examiner may pass to the next sextant.

The management of patients according to their sextant scores is suggested below:

Code 0:
No treatment.

Code 1:
OHI.

Code 2:
OHI plus removal of calculus and correction of plaque retentive margins or fillings or crowns. Patients whose CPITN score for all sextants are Codes 0, 1, 2 should be screened again after an interval of one year.

Code 3:
As Code 2 but a longer time will be required for treatment. Plaque and bleeding scores are collected at the start and finish of treatment.
    Probing depths in the sextants scoring Code 3 will be taken at the finish of treatment.
    Subsequently these records should be taken at intervals of not more than one year along with CPITN screening of other sextants.

*Code 4: or Code *
A full probing depth chart is required, together with recordings of gingival recession, furcation involvement and any other relevant clinical details. Individual intraoral radiographs will be taken of teeth which show furcation involvement or loss of attachment of 7 mm or more at any site.
    Treatment will include oral hygiene instruction, removal of calculus and overhangs and root planing.
    Re-examination is then required to assess the results of treatment to date and the need for further treatment which may include periodontal surgery.

Practitioners may wish to refer patients with scores 4 or * for specialist care.

This is a screening system and is not intended to be used for monitoring purposes during treatment. Readers are referred to the policy document for recording and monitoring methods suited to this purpose.

Classification of Periodontal Diseases

EXPLANATORY NOTES

The classification below describes in a simple form the inter-relationships of different forms of periodontal disease. It is based on a classification described by Ramfjord and Ash (1979).

Plaque-associated diseases have an inflammatory basis with bacterial plaque as the primary aetiological agent.

Simple gingivitis is the common form of chronic gingivitis where no unusual modifying factors are present. Complex gingivitis occurs when specific local or systemic modifying factors exist.

Simple periodontitis is a slowly progressive disease usually found in adults but which may have its onset in adolescence. Complex periodontitis is a rapidly destructive form of periodontal disease where there is a major imbalance between the micro-organisms and the host response. It is usually classified by age of onset. Complex adult periodontitis, unlike prepubertal and juvenile periodontitis, is not well characterised and may be described in contemporary literature as 'rapidly progressive', 'postjuvenile', 'advanced destructive' or 'severe' periodontitis, etc. 'Rapidly progressive' and 'postjuvenile' periodontitis are terms usually applied only to young adult dentitions, although rapid loss of attachment may also affect middle-aged and elderly individuals. Until the means exists to identify a 'burst' of destructive activity as it occurs, obtaining a diagnosis of the exact *type* of periodontitis (something which can be done only in retrospect) will not be important to the *clinician*. All periodontitis, and indeed gingivitis, should be regarded as potentially harmful and treated accordingly.

Non-plaque-associated diseases may occur independently or concurrently with plaque-associated diseases. Pathological processes, other than those listed, may affect the periodontal tissue but are not normally considered as forms of periodontal disease. These conditions include neoplasia, renal osteodystrophy, scleroderma and hyperparathyroidism.

CLASSIFICATION

A. Plaque-associated Diseases

a) Gingivitis
   i) Chronic
      Simple gingivitis
      Complex gingivitis
      e.g. mouth-breathing gingivitis
            pregnancy gingivitis
            leukaemic gingivitis
            puberty gingivitis
            phenytoin hyperplasia
            hereditary gingival fibromatosis
   ii) Acute
      Necrotising ulcerative gingivitis
      Gingival abscess
b) Periodontitis
   i) Chronic
      Simple periodontitis
      Complex periodontitis
      e.g. complex adult periodontitis
            juvenile periodontitis
            prepubertal periodontitis
   ii) Acute
      Periodontal abscess

B. Non-plaque-associated Diseases

a) Traumatic
      Occlusal trauma
      Traumatic gingival recession
b) Infective
      Acute herpetic stomatitis
c) Dermatological
      Desquamative gingivitis

REFERENCE

Ramfjord S. P., Ash M. M., Jr. (1979). Classification and epidemiology of periodontal diseases. In *Periodontology and Periodontics*. Ch. 6. Eastbourne: W. B. Saunders.

Index